MW00763204

Neurological Disorders and Imaging Physics, Volume 1

Application of multiple sclerosis

Ed elli a me: 'Ritorna a tua scïenza,
che vuol, quanto la cosa è più perfetta,
più senta il bene, e così la doglienza.'

(And he to me: 'the more a thing is perfect,
the more keenly it will feel
both pleasure and pain.')

Dante Alighieri, Italian poet (1265–1321)
Divine Comedy,
Canto VI, lines 106–108

The most beautiful thing we can experience is the mysterious. It is the source of all true art and science.

Albert Einstein, physicist (1879–1955)

Neurological Disorders and Imaging Physics, Volume 1

Application of multiple sclerosis

Luca Saba
Department of Radiology, AOU of Cagliari, Italy

Jasjit S Suri
AtheroPoint, CA, USA

IOP Publishing, Bristol, UK

ISBN 978-0-7503-1759-7 (ebook)
ISBN 978-0-7503-1757-3 (print)
ISBN 978-0-7503-1758-0 (mobi)

DOI 10.1088/2053-2563/ab1fdc

Version: 20191001

IOP ebooks
ISSN 2053-2563 (online)
ISSN 2054-7315 (print)

British Library Cataloguing-in-Publication Data: A catalogue record for this book is available from the British Library.

Published by IOP Publishing, wholly owned by The Institute of Physics, London

IOP Publishing, Temple Circus, Temple Way, Bristol, BS1 6HG, UK

US Office: IOP Publishing, Inc., 190 North Independence Mall West, Suite 601, Philadelphia, PA 19106, USA

This book is dedicated to my students, residents and fellows as a way of thanking them for what they have taught me.

Contents

Preface

Owing to its ability to depict the pathologic features of multiple sclerosis (MS) in exquisite detail, conventional magnetic resonance imaging (MRI) has become an established tool in the diagnosis of this disease and in monitoring its evolution. MRI has been formally included in the diagnostic work-up of patients who present with a clinically isolated syndrome suggestive of MS, and ad hoc diagnostic criteria have been proposed and are updated on a regular basis. Over the past few decades, MRI-based visualization of demyelinated CNS lesions has become pivotal to the diagnosis and monitoring of MS.

In the last few years, newer MRI technologies, including higher-field-strength MR units, have been developed to estimate the overall multiple sclerosis burden and mechanisms of recovery in patients at different stages of the disease.

The purpose of this book is to cover all the imaging techniques and new exciting methods for the analysis of MS with the most world renowned scientists in these fields.

Luca Saba and Jasjit S Suri
Cagliari, Italy, 26 April 2019

Acknowledgements

It is not possible to overstate my gratitude to the many individuals who helped to produce this book. I would like to thank my colleagues at the University of Cagliari for interesting discussions about advanced imaging and Paolo Siotto for continuous support and many suggestions. A special thanks to my wife, Tiziana—without your continuous encouragement this book would not have been completed, I have to say that this is also your book! Thank you for your great work.

Luca Saba
Cagliari, Italy, 26 April 2019

Editor biographies

Luca Saba

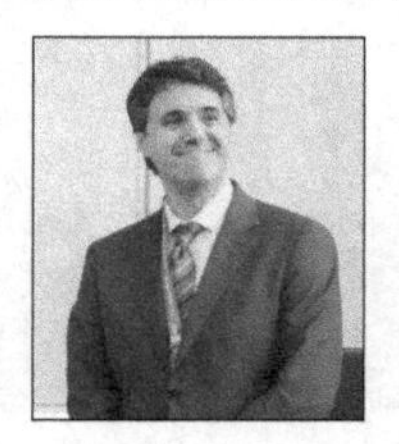

Luca Saba is a Full Professor of Radiology and Chief of the Department of Radiology at the AOU of Cagliari. Professor Saba's research is focused on multi-detector-row computed tomography, magnetic resonance, ultrasound, neuroradiology and diagnosis in vascular sciences.

His work has, as lead author, led to more than 300 publications in high-impact-factor, peer-reviewed journals, such as *Lancet Neurology*, *Radiology*, *American Journal of Neuroradiology*, *Atherosclerosis*, *European Radiology*, *European Journal of Radiology*, *Acta Radiologica*, *Cardiovascular and Interventional Radiology*, *Journal of Computer Assisted Tomography*, *American Journal of Roentgenology*, *Neuroradiology*, *Clinical Radiology*, *Journal of Cardiovascular Surgery*, *Cerebrovascular Diseases*, *Brain Pathology*, *Medical Physics* and *Atherosclerosis*. He is a well known speaker and has spoken over 70 times at national and international levels.

Dr Saba has won 15 scientific and extracurricular awards during his career. He has presented more than 500 papers and posters at national and international conferences (RSNA, ESGAR, ECR, ISR, AOCR, AINR, JRS, SIRM and AINR). He has written 21 book-chapters and is the editor of 14 books in the fields of computed tomography, cardiovascular disease, plastic surgery, gynecological imaging and neurodegenerative imaging.

He is member of the Italian Society of Radiology (SIRM), European Society of Radiology (ESR), Radiological Society of North America (RSNA), American Roentgen Ray Society (ARRS), Italian Association of Neuroradiology (AINR), International Society for Magnetic Resonance in Medicine (ISMRM), American Society of Functional Neuroradiology (ASFNR) and European Society of Neuroradiology (ESNR), and serves as a reviewer for more than 50 scientific journals.

Jasjit S Suri

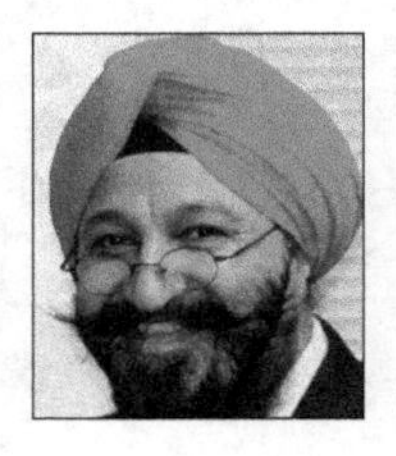

Dr Jasjit S Suri, PhD, MBA, Fellow of AIMBE, is an innovator, visionary, scientist and an internationally known world leader in his field. Dr Suri received the Director General's Gold Medal in 1980 and became a Fellow of the American Institute of Medical and Biological Engineering, awarded by the National Academy of Sciences, Washington, DC, in 2004. In 2018, Dr Suri received the Marquis Life Time Achievement Award. He is currently Chairman of AtheroPoint, Roseville, CA, USA, a company dedicated to atherosclerosis imaging for early screening of stroke and cardiovascular disease.

List of contributors

Roberto Scipione
University of Roma la Sapienza

Andrea Leonardi
University of Roma la Sapienza

Fabrizio Andrani
University of Roma la Sapienza

Carola Palla
University of Roma la Sapienza

Arianna Sanna
University of Roma la Sapienza

Michele Anzidei
University of Roma la Sapienza

Michele Porcu
University of Cagliari

Antonella Balestrieri
University of Cagliari

Paolo Garofalo
University of Cagliari

Luigi Barberini
University of Cagliari

Paolo Siotto
AOB Cagliari

James T Grist
University of Birmingham

Frank Riemer
Cambridge University

Tomasz Matys
Cambridge University

Rhys Slough
Cambridge University

Fulvio Zaccagna
Cambridge University

Giuseppe Corrias
University of Cagliari

Gian Carlo Coghe
University of Cagliari

Giuseppe Fenu
University of Cagliari

Jessica Frau
University of Cagliari

Lorena Lorefice
University of Cagliari

Eleonora Cocco
University of Cagliari

Francesco Destro
University of Cagliari

Gerardo Dessì
ATS Sardegna

Vincenzo Secchi
ATS Sardegna

Maria Elisabetta Barraccu
ATS Sardegna

Thanis Saksirinukul
University of Bangkok

Chapter 1

Magnetic resonance imaging

Roberto Scipione, Andrea Leonardi, Fabrizio Andrani, Carola Palla, Arianna Sanna and Michele Anzidei

Magnetic resonance (MR) plays a leading role in neurological imaging, providing optimal identification of anatomic structures and also allowing the evaluation of functional and chemical aspects of both the central and peripheral nervous systems.

These tools have increased the comprehension of different neurological disorders and improved the evaluation of treatment response to pharmacological or other therapeutic interventions. Moreover, several innovative MR techniques, such as functional magnetic resonance imaging (fMRI), MR spectroscopy (MRS) and diffusion-weighted imaging (DWI), have been shown to provide additional information, allowing a comprehensive evaluation in the identification of a wide range of nervous system pathologies.

However, body MRI may also be useful to depict several causes and manifestations of neurological pathologies, thus supporting a multidisciplinary diagnosis process.

In this chapter, a brief discussion of MR basics will be presented, with particular attention on the aspects related to the evaluation of neurological disorders.

1.1 Introduction

Magnetic resonance (MR) plays a leading role in neurological imaging, providing optimal identification of anatomic structures and also allowing the evaluation of functional and chemical aspects in both the central and peripheral nervous systems. These tools have increased our comprehension of different neurological disorders and improved the evaluation of treatment response to pharmacological or other therapeutic interventions. Moreover, several innovative MR techniques, such as functional magnetic resonance imaging (fMRI), MR spectroscopy (MRS) and diffusion-weighted imaging (DWI), have been demonstrated to provide additional information, allowing a comprehensive evaluation in the identification of a wide range of nervous system pathologies. In particular, MRI has become an established

doi:10.1088/2053-2563/ab1fdcch1

tool in the diagnosis of multiple sclerosis (MS) and other demyelinating diseases and in monitoring their evolution, thanks to its ability to depict the pathological features in exquisite detail.

Moreover, the introduction of MR and the continuous technological innovation behind new tools, sequences and other elements, have allowed the comprehension of a wide range of other neurological disorders, demonstrating connections between the most various anatomic and functional alterations. At the same time, body MRI may be useful to depict several causes and manifestations of neurological pathologies, thus supporting a multidisciplinary diagnostic process.

In this chapter, a brief discussion of MR basics will be presented, with particular attention on the aspects related to the evaluation of neurological disorders.

1.2 Magnetic resonance imaging

1.2.1 General physical principles

Magnetic resonance imaging (MRI) is based on the physical features of hydrogen atoms or protons (H^+) embedded in water molecules and their magnetic dipoles. Under the influence of external magnetic fields, these protons produce electrical signals [1, 2] that can be recorded by specific tools; the application of a specific spatial coding procedure allows the signal to be processed in order to obtain the final diagnostic images.

The entire process requires: a magnet, providing a constant magnetic field (B_0); a system of gradients, providing orthogonal fields for spatial localization of signal; a radiofrequency (RF) system, with transmitter coils providing additional fields for spin excitation; and receiver coils, receiving MR signal over the imaging volume.

When a volume is put inside a field B_0, all the vectors that describe the magnetization of each proton are aligned. After the application of an RF set, the H^+ are flipped out of their alignment and start precessing with the same phase. From this moment, up to the point where the perturbed H^+ come back to their previous aligned state (relaxation) [3], an electric signal can be obtained by specific receiving coils. The simultaneous application of gradient magnets ensures this process occurs only in a slice of the whole volume of interest. Further spatial coding provides the location of protons in the exact voxel within that slice.

The whole process requires specific MRI protocol settings, with a whole set of parameters that can be customized according to the specific diagnostic needs, including the characteristics of the RF pulse, echo time (TE), repetition time (TR), matrix, field of view (FOV) and flip angles (FAs). TE represents the time between RF excitation and first acquisition of the signal, while TR is the time interval between subsequent RF excitations. The variation of TR and TE determines the modification of the contrast of the image, reflecting different properties of tissues in terms of longitudinal magnetization recovery (T1) and transverse magnetization decay (T2). In particular, long TR and TE lead to T2-weighted imaging, while short TR and TE lead to T1-weighted imaging. Each MR signal decodes for intensity, spatial and phase information; the different signal information is collected in the so-called k-space, which can be subsequently converted into a readable image by using a mathematical process (two-dimensional Fourier transform).

A pulse sequence indicates a determinate series of RF waves and electromagnetic gradients, administrated in order to create MR images. Pulse sequences are basically classified into two families, spin echo (SE) sequences and gradient echo (GE) sequences.

A typical SE sequence requires a 90° followed by a 180° RF pulse, whereas GE sequences are characterized by a lack of the refocusing 180° RF pulse and a flip angle (FA) equal to or smaller than 90°. Among specific sequences, it is worth mentioning echo-planar imaging (EPI) sequences, which represent the basis for several advanced techniques that will be covered in this chapter, such as DTI and fMRI. A dedicated MRI study of the brain can include, beyond conventional sequences, advanced imaging sequences, such as fMRI, MRS, ASL, DTI, with special reference to the individual clinical case.

1.2.2 Conventional MR sequences

All conventional MR images derive from classical SE and GE pulse sequences. The basis of conventional MR imaging in neurological disorders is to depict anatomy, to detect pathological variants or abnormalities, and to emphasize specific morphological changes in the tissue structure. The use of paramagnetic contrast agent (in TSE or GE sequences) represents another useful tool that may provide further information in the whole diagnostic process.

Conventional MR sequences, with and without administration of a contrast agent, provide important pieces of information for diagnosing MS, understanding its natural history and assessing treatment efficacy. Some of these sequences show the highest sensitivity for detection of MS lesions, but also have low specificity, due to a low ability to differentiate areas of abnormal signal coming from different pathological alterations that might be present (even at the same time) in the natural history of the disease, such as edema, inflammation, demyelination, remyelination, gliosis and axonal loss.

1.2.2.1 Spin echo sequences

SE sequences are obtained by a fundamental sequence of 90°–180° RF pulses (figure 1.1). Modifying TR and TE, it is possible to highlight specific characteristics for each tissue, obtaining T1-weighted and T2-weighted images. As previously described, short TR and short TE (less than 700 and 30 ms, respectively) highlight the differences in T1 properties between tissues (T1-weighting), while long TE and TR (greater than 2000 and 80 ms, respectively) highlight the differences in T2 properties between tissues (T2 weighting). Long TR and short TE highlight the differences of proton density between tissues, minimizing the T1-weighted and the T2-weighted contrast of the image.

Due to their long acquisition time, these classical sequences are actually less used. Advances in MR technology have introduced innovative fast SE sequences, reducing the acquisition time. In a fast SE (FSE) or turbo SE (TSE) sequence, a single 90°

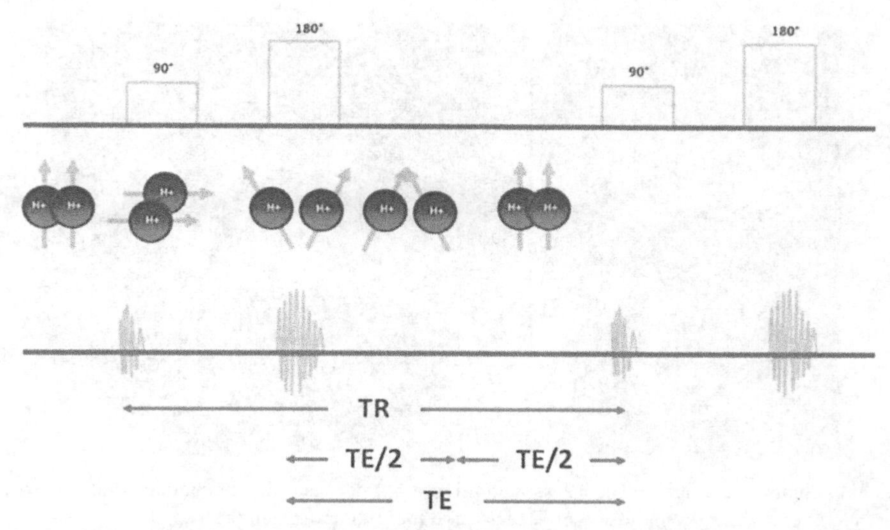

Figure 1.1. Schematic representation of an SE sequence displaying radiofrequency pulses and corresponding proton excitement. TR: time of repetition. TE: time of echo.

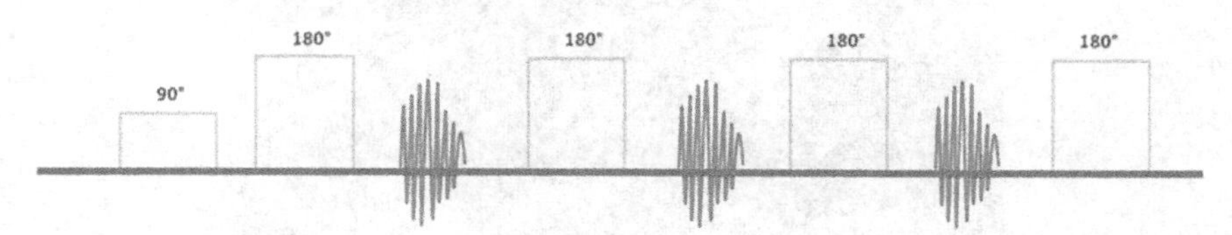

Figure 1.2. Schematic representation of a fast spin echo (FSE) sequence. The echo train is composed of a series of sequential 180° pulses, permitting the acquisition of multiple lines of volume for each TR, thus allowing an overall shorter imaging time.

pulse is applied to flip the net magnetization vector, after which multiple 180° rephasing pulses are applied (echo train, figure 1.2). The main use of TSE sequences is to acquire T2-w images, due to the significant reduction in scan time that can be achieved for long TR scans when modest echo train lengths are used. TSE sequences can also be applied to produce T1-w images.

Echo train lengths less than ten are typically used for brain and spine imaging, but very long echo trains (100 or more) can be used in abdominal imaging to acquire T2-weighted images in less than one second. These classic sequences (SE or TSE) with different weighting (T1, T2 or PD), allow one to depict several causes and manifestations of neurological disorders—local or diffuse, acute or chronic—often allowing a specific diagnosis to be obtained without any further diagnostic assessment (figures 1.3 and 1.4).

1.2.2.2 Gradient echo sequences

In contrast to standard SE sequences, that use a 180° pulse to refocus the protons with a longer time of acquisition, GE sequences (figure 1.5) are shorter, since they employ gradient reversal pulses in at least two directions to generate the echo signal.

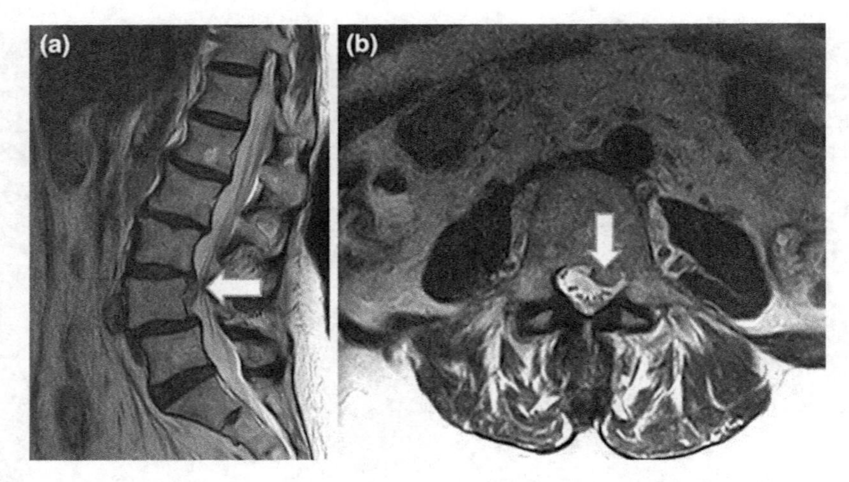

Figure 1.3. Lumbar disc hernia. The T2-w sagittal image (a) depicts a disc herniation (white arrows), with caudal migration, causing compression of left L4 nerve root at dural origin (b).

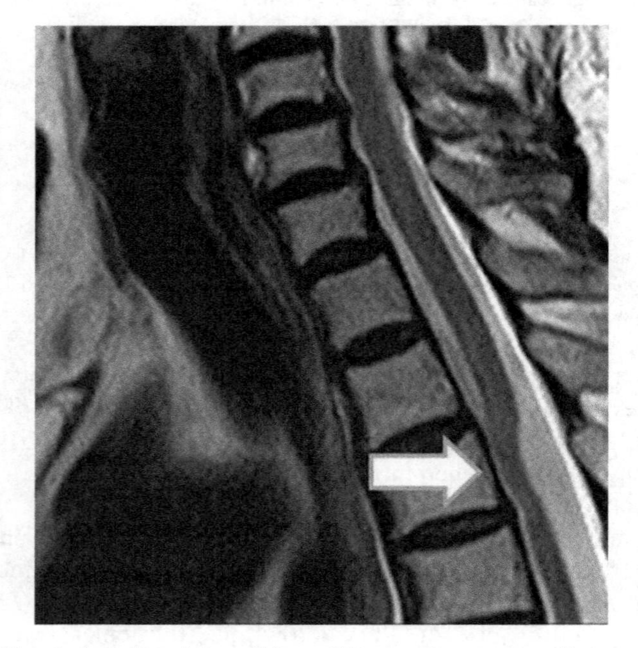

Figure 1.4. Idiopathic spinal cord herniation. This condition is only encountered between T2 and T8, where the normal thoracic kyphosis leads to the thoracic cord being in close proximity to the ventral theca. The key feature is focal distortion and rotation of the cord with no CSF seen between it and the ventral theca (as well demonstrated on this T2-w image, white arrow).

The main advantage of GE sequences is represented by their short TR (which reflects a faster time of acquisition). However, the principles behind GE techniques also have some disadvantages. For example, the absence of the 180° refocus pulse causes a lower efficiency at reducing magnetic inhomogeneity, with consequent more

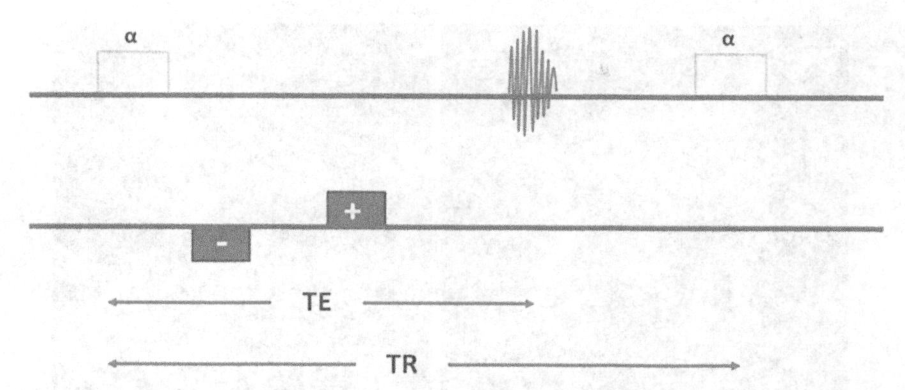

Figure 1.5. Schematic representation of a GE sequence. Slice-selective gradients are employed with limited flip angles (about 45°). Dephasing and rephrasing of transverse magnetization are determined by alternating negative phase-encoding and positive frequency-encoding gradients.

consistent loss in the precession phase among protons, that is reflected by a lower signal-to-noise ratio (SNR) and lower anatomic detail in the final image. In fact, the faster loss of phase determines a faster loss of transversal magnetization, that is described by a specific weighting called T2*, particularly sensitive and susceptible to magnetic field inhomogeneity, that may be induced by the presence of some substances such as air, calcium or iron. Because of these features, GE sequences have a primary role in neuroimaging for the evaluation of hemorrhages and other causes of iron deposition. In particular, iron deposition may also be observed in MS, due to the inflammatory process that causes multiple effects, such as the interruption of the blood–brain barrier, accumulation of iron-rich macrophages, reduced axonal clearance of iron and iron-induced neurodegeneration.

Coherent or partially refocused GRE sequences use a gradient to maintain the T2* and eventually produce T2-w images. The fundamental difference between partially refocused and fully refocused GRE sequences is that all the gradients in the latter are refocused. In contrast, incoherent or spoiled GRE sequences utilize, after each echo, a specific RF pulse or gradient, called a spoiler, to null the T2* effect, thereby producing T1 or proton density weighting. Partially refocused GRE images are mostly used in imaging of encephalic nerves and internal auditory canal structures (figure 1.6), while spoiled GRE sequences are widely employed in contrast-enhanced MRI.

Steady state free precession (SSFP) represents a specific fully rephased GE technique, with continuous repetition of short TRs (5 ms). SSFP guarantees the best temporal resolution among MR pulse sequences and a high SNR, but also extreme susceptibility to artifacts caused by magnetic field inhomogeneities. These sequences are employed in cardiovascular and gastroenteric imaging, due to the high signal achieved from blood vessels and static fluids.

1.2.2.3 Fat and fluid signal suppression

MRI allows the selective suppression of the signal of specific tissues (saturation). This tool is widely used to achieve a better characterization during the diagnostic

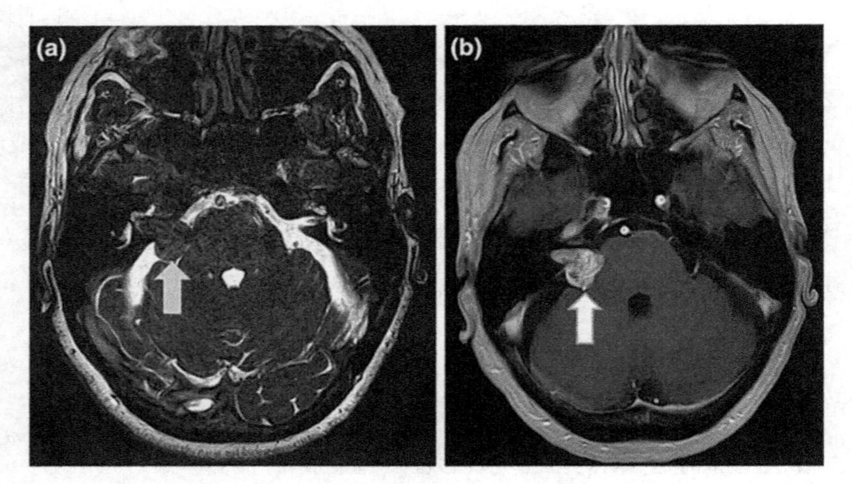

Figure 1.6. Acoustic neuroma. This lesion is classically present on imaging as a solid nodular mass with an intracanalicular component that often results in widening of the porus acusticus, as well demonstrated by this constructive interference in steady state (CISS; yellow arrow) sequence (a) and confirmed by a T1 post-Gd sequence (white arrow) (b).

process. The most common structures that are suppressed during MRI include fat, cerebrospinal fluid and silicon.

Fat saturation allows easy identification of lesions contacting adipocytes or intracytoplasmic fat, but it is advantageous even in order to enhance signal from other tissues, silencing the 'fat background' (e.g. in the identification of edema). Several methods for fat saturation can be used in MRI. The most common method is applying a frequency-selective saturation RF pulse or spoiler gradient to null the fat signal, immediately subsequent to the 90° initial pulse. This strategy is fast, specific for fat and can be used with any imaging sequences, in particular in contrast-enhanced MRI. On the other hand, it is burdened by artifacts due to magnetic field inhomogeneities and incomplete suppression.

The second method is inversion recovery (IR) imaging, obtained with the application of an initial 180° pulse, to flip the net magnetization vector of fat tissue; if the 90° pulse is applied in the exact fat 'null interval' (140 ms), a suppression of fat signal is obtained (STIR, short tau inversion recovery) (figure 1.7). STIR sequences are widely used in MR protocols in order to detect solid lesions, as well as edema due to traumatic, functional or vascular injuries. This technique requires long acquisition duration, because of its long TR.

The third strategy is so-called 'out-of-phase imaging'. This technique takes advantage of the different precession rates between protons in fat (CH_2) and water (H_2O), using spoiled GRE sequences—in those voxels where CH_2 and H_2O are present in the same proportion, the signal is nulled. It is important to point out that this technique enables the saturation of 'microscopical fat' (steroids or triglycerides deposits), characteristically present in adenomatous cells and steatosis hepatocytes.

In the field of neurological disorders, suppression of cerebrospinal fluid (CSF) signal (obtained with fluid-attenuated inversion recovery (FLAIR)) plays a

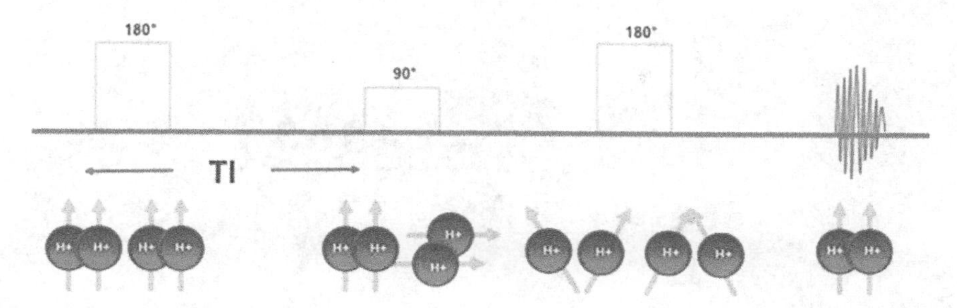

Figure 1.7. Schematic representation of an STIR sequence. A 180° nulling RP is employed to suppress fat or water signals. After a determined inversion time (TI) at the fat 'null interval', a 90° pulse is applied to start the usual SE sequence.

fundamental role, with particular application to MS and other demyelination disorders. Silencing the CSF signal allows the identification of demyelinating plaques with critical locations, such as those adjacent to cortical sulci or ventricles, that might not be distinguished otherwise due to the low contrast with CSF. The FLAIR sequence also allows the evaluation of edema in the central nervous system, a signal of tissue damage from vascular causes or compression from a growing mass.

The principle of inversion recovery can also be potentially extended to any tissue by knowing the specific relaxation time of that tissue. For example, a promising sequence that has been recently introduced in the evaluation of MS is double-inversion-recovery, which uses two inversion times to suppress the signal from both white matter and CSF, in order to provide a better identification of cortical and other gray matter locations that are typically not seen in conventional MR studies.

1.2.2.4 Proton density

As mentioned above, long TRs (2000–5000 ms) and short TEs (10–20 ms) determine the silencing of T1- and T2-weighted contrast among different tissues in the diagnostic image; in this case higher signal is obtained by structures with higher density of protons (proton density (PD) sequence).

PD sequences are still used in neuroimaging, even if their application currently plays a secondary role due to the introduction of more recent techniques such as FLAIR sequences that have shown more accurate results in highlighting the contrast between CSF and lesions located in proximity to cortical sulci or ventricles. However, PD sequences are still widely adopted in musculoskeletal imaging protocols, since they allow an accurate evaluation of cartilage.

1.2.2.5 Echo-planar imaging

In this technique, available for both SE and GRE sequences, a single echo train is employed to acquire the entire volume, with a consequent very short acquisition time. In fact, in echo-planar imaging (EPI), multiple lines of data are acquired after a single RF excitation (single-shot EPI) or more RF pulses (multi-shot EPI). The latter guarantees higher spatial resolution and reduction of image distortion and signal loss due to susceptibility differences, T2 relaxation and main field

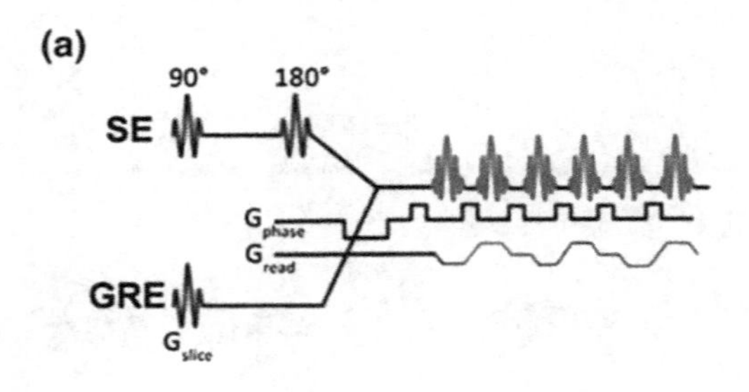

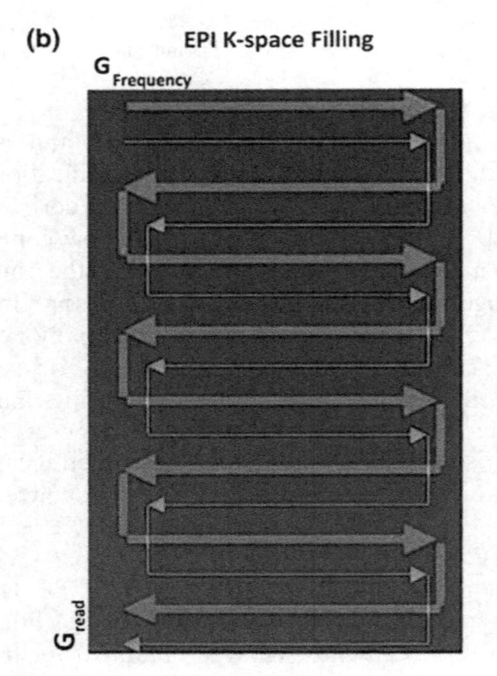

Figure 1.8. (a) Schematic representation of an echo-planar imaging sequence, for both SE and GRE sequences, with phase-encoding and frequency-encoding gradients rapidly turned on and off in order to shorten acquisition time. (b) Corresponding k-space filling geometry in EPI.

inhomogeneities [4]. Echo-planar imaging is now a technique of choice for diffusion-weighted imaging (figure 1.8).

1.2.3 Contrast-enhanced MRI

Contrast-enhanced MRI (CE-MRI) is based on the principle of shortening the T1 relaxation of tissues through the intravenous injection of Gd-chelate contrast agents. In the evaluation of neurological disorders, it is important to point out that an increase in signal intensity after contrast agent injection does not indicate a higher vascularization of tissues, but rather damage or interruption of the ematoencephalic barrier. Specifically, in the assessment of demyelinating processes, CE-MRI allows the distinction between active and inactive lesions, since enhancement occurs as a result of increased ematoencephalic barrier permeability and corresponds to areas of ongoing inflammation.

Moreover, plaques that persistently appear dark on pre- and post-contrast T1-weighted images ('black holes') are associated with axonal loss, indicating a more severe tissue damage.

The CE-MRI technique gives no quantitative insight into hemodynamic processes, thus many dynamic contrast-enhanced (DCE) techniques have been designed, in order to provide further help in differential diagnosis of pathological processes. The principal perfusional imaging technique is based on gadolinium bolus injection and subsequent acquisition of T1-weighted gradient echo sequence with short TE (<1.5 ms) and TR (<7 ms) and a flip angle around 30° [5]. Because of the very short acquisition time, these sequences can be sequentially obtained at several time points after the injection of the contrast agent in order to quantitatively evaluate contrast medium extraction, thanks to a wide range of parameters obtained by pharmacokinetic modeling, such as transfer constant (K_{trans}) and fractional volume of the interstitial space (v_e). A color map can be also obtained from these parameters, to display the perfusion and permeability of tissues. The K_{trans} assessed in the first pass of contrast medium indicates a high barrier permeability, while that measured at the steady state better describes lower permeability, when K_{trans} is dependent on surface area and is not flow limited.

Many studies have applied DCE-MRI in the detection and characterization of neoplasms in many regions [6, 7], with great attention on CNS malignancy [8].

1.2.4 Magnetic resonance angiography (MRA)

Magnetic resonance angiography (MRA) has become one of the fundamental imaging modalities in the management of vascular pathologies, even in the evaluation of neurological disorders [9, 10]. MR angiographic sequences can be performed with or without contrast medium injection. Time-of-flight (TOF) and phase-contrast (PC) MRA are non-contrast techniques that can detect the signal coming from intravascular blood due to its movement compared to static tissues. Contrast-enhanced (CE) MRA relies on the T1 shortening effect of intravenously administered contrast medium circulating in the blood.

In TOF-MRA, saturation of stationary tissues is obtained by a series of RF pulses with a repetition time much shorter than tissue T1 values, 'silencing' the vector of longitudinal magnetization [11]. At the same time, inflowing unsaturated blood still has a large longitudinal magnetization vector, so it will be seen in the imaged slice as an area of high signal intensity [12]. However, intravascular flowing protons are also subject to saturation effects that are proportional to the time these protons stay in the slice of interest. Therefore, short TR, slow flow and the course of the blood vessel in the imaging slice plane all unfavorably affect vessel-to-background contrast.

TOF-MRA can be either performed by acquiring sequential, independent slices (2D TOF-MRA) or by acquiring a volume that is subsequently partitioned into separate slices (3D TOF-MRA).

Currently, the main application of TOF-MRA (particularly using 3D sequences) regards the study of intracranial arterial circulation. In this context, TOF provides the visualization of major intracranial arteries and peripheral branches in a relatively short time and without any contrast agent, allowing the diagnosis of pathological conditions, such as stenosis or intracranial aneurysm (figure 1.9). On the other hand, the application of TOF-MRA in other anatomical districts is limited by the long duration of acquisition, a tendency for stenosis overestimation and different types of artifacts (motion artifacts, ghosting, flow void). However, it could be a useful back-up modality in patients who cannot receive contrast medium.

Phase-contrast (PC)-MRA represents another non-contrast MRA technique, that generates vascular contrast following a different approach compared to TOF-MRA. This technique generates vessel-to-background contrast by displaying the accumulated phase difference in terms of transverse magnetization between moving and stationary protons [13]. PC acquisition is more sensitive to slow flows, such as in venous vessels.

As previously mentioned, CE-MRA is based on the differences in the T1 relaxation times of blood and surrounding tissues when a rapid bolus infusion of a paramagnetic contrast agent is injected [14]. These gadolinium-based agents exert a T1 shortening effect, generating a high intravascular SNR, which is largely unaffected by inflow.

Signal intensity (i.e. T1-weighted shortening) within the target vessel obviously depends on the amount of gadolinium within the vascular bed at the moment of acquisition. Therefore, imaging should be ideally performed at the peak of vascular

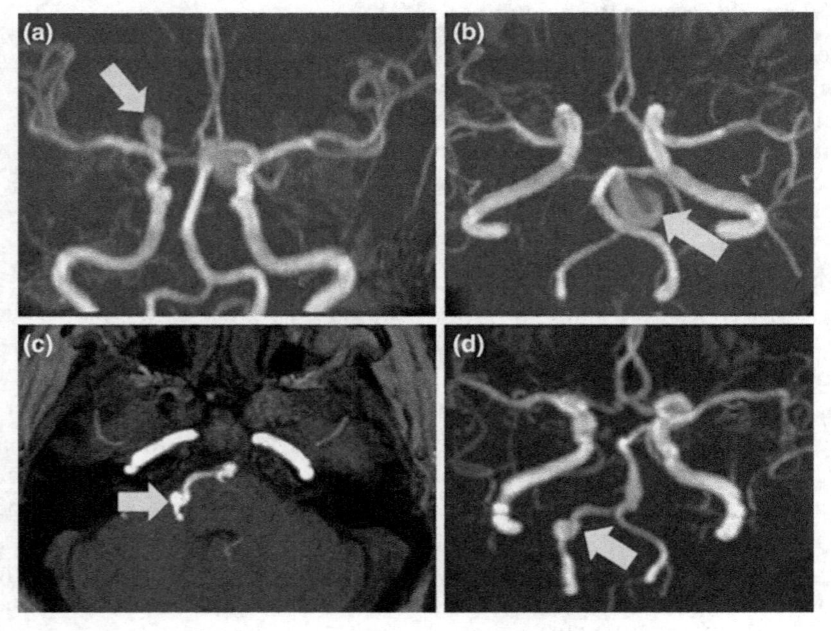

Figure 1.9. TOF-MRA for the study of intracranial aneurysms in several localities: right middle cerebral artery (a), basilar artery, with signs of rupture (b), and right vertebral artery (c), (d).

enhancement, when a maximum difference exists between the signal intensity of the target vessel and the surrounding overlapping structures [15]. Unlike TOF and PC imaging, the signal of vessels in CE-MRA is based on the intrinsic T1 signal of blood, rather than flow effects. Therefore, as already mentioned above, this technique is less flow sensitive, which means that the image quality is not degraded by the numerous flow-related artifacts that may occur during acquisition, such as signal loss from spin saturation, or slow-flow phenomena potentially mimicking a significant stenosis or vascular occlusion, particularly in vessels with relatively small caliber, such as carotid arteries.

A further relevant advantage of CE-MRA is that the usual loss of SNR from faster scanning can be compensated by injecting the same dose of contrast faster over a shorter scan duration. In this way, faster scanning can attain higher-quality images with fewer motion artifacts. With CE-MRA, the pause between arterial enhancement and the onset of venous enhancement (i.e. arteriovenous window) offers an opportunity for arterial phase imaging that shows only the arteries.

A practical aspect of CE-MRA to consider is the vessel-to-background contrast. The T1 decrease in the vessel, due to contrast medium injection, is not sufficient to selectively enhance arteries and to suppress background tissue. As a result, the signal of these tissues—and specifically, fat tissue—must be eliminated to present easily understandable images. The most commonly used technique is subtraction of non-enhanced 'mask' images, identical to the 3D CE-MRA volumes.

All these features make this technique an important diagnostic tool in the management of patients with vasculature symptoms, with the aim to recognize or characterize pathological findings responsible for neurological disorders.

1.2.5 Diffusion-weight imaging (DWI)

Diffusion-weighted imaging (DWI) is an MRI technique based on differences in Brownian random motion of water molecules between tissues, reflecting histological organization [16].

DWI uses either an echo-planar or a fast GRE sequence in order to distinguish between unrestricted diffusion (rapid diffusion of protons) and restricted diffusion (slow diffusion of protons). The main disadvantages of this technique are represented by its low resolution, low SNR and high sensitivity to physiological motion.

Single-shot echo-planar imaging (EPI) is commonly preferred to reduce motion sensitivity. The design of these sequences requires a pair of large gradient pulses placed on both sides of the 180° refocusing pulse; the first gradient pulse dephases the magnetization across the voxel, while the second pulse rephases the magnetization. For stationary (non-diffusing) molecules, the phases induced by both gradients will completely cancel, and there will be no signal attenuation from diffusion. On the other hand, in the case of net movement, protons are not affected by both gradients (they may undergo dephasing but not rephasing, or vice versa), and therefore there is a decrease in signal intensity. Signal loss is directly proportional to the degree of water motion along the same direction of the diffusion gradient, while no signal loss occurs if the motion is perpendicular to the gradient direction.

The gradient strength is expressed in terms of the *b*-value. This factor is proportional to the diffusion time interval and the square of the strength of the diffusion gradient. A larger *b*-value is achieved by increasing the gradient amplitude and duration and by widening the interval between paired gradient pulses. The detection of slow-moving water molecules and smaller diffusion distances requires higher *b*-values (e.g. $b = 550 \text{ s mm}^{-2}$). All diffusion images should be compared with a reference image, such as a standard SE image, in which the strength of the diffusion gradient is zero.

When describing DWI techniques, it is important also to consider the complementary ADC map. In fact, even if stringent measures have been taken to avoid the effects of gross motion and flow, a diffusion-weighted image is still affected by MR properties other than diffusion, e.g. T2 weighting. To remove all effects other than diffusion, it is mandatory to use the apparent diffusion coefficient, as described. In order to obtain an image of the ADC values, two acquisitions are necessary: one set obtained without application of a diffusion gradient (which has an appearance similar to that of T2-weighted images), and one obtained with a diffusion gradient. The ADC calculation takes into account those two sets of images, in order to differentiate a real diffusion restriction phenomenon from a 'T2 shine-through' artifact (which is due to a high T2 signal which 'shines through' to the DWI images even at higher *b*-values). In clinical neurological practice, the absence of corresponding effects on ADC maps allows areas of restricted diffusion from a recent stroke to appear dark and areas of unrestricted diffusion from an older stroke to appear relatively bright. Therefore, DWI has always to be evaluated in comparison with ADC maps, in order to allow the determination of the age of a stroke.

The visualization of changes in the diffusion properties of tissue water with MR imaging has become a useful tool to characterize tissue structure and to identify and differentiate disease processes. DWI is routinely used in investigations of stroke in brain imaging [17] and has also obtained an important role in oncologic imaging, in which it may indicate tumor cellularity.

1.2.6 Diffusion tensor imaging

Diffusion tensor imaging (DTI) is an extension of DWI that is based on white matter (WM) tract orientation. In fact, diffusion of water molecules follows the 'pathway of least resistance' along the direction of WM fibers. In order to obtain a final diagnostic image from this feature, DTI considers anisotropic diffusion to estimate the axonal (WM) organization of the brain. Collected data can be further processed in order to obtain 3D reconstruction of neural tracts, known as fiber tractography (FT).

Since axonal membranes and myelin sheaths represent barriers to the motion of water molecules in directions not parallel to their own orientation, diffusion is 'anisotropic' (directionally dependent) in WM fiber tracts, meaning that the direction of maximum diffusivity coincides with WM fiber tract orientation [18]. The diffusion tensor is a mathematical model of diffusion in three-dimensional space that describes the magnitude, the degree of anisotropy and the orientation of diffusion anisotropy. In this way, the diffusion tensor allows the identification of mutual connections between different functional centers and highlights any possible alterations due to pathological situations [19], including demyelination and axonal loss due to and other demyelinating diseases.

In order to calculate the diffusion tensor, it is mandatory to acquire at least six diffusion gradients and the corresponding ADC maps along six orthogonal directions (three orthogonal, x, y, z, and three combined, xy, xz, yz). Using more than six encoding directions will improve the accuracy of the tensor measurement for any arbitrary orientation [20]. When assessing a diffusion tensor protocol, the determination of the optimum b-value is complicated by the involvement of many factors, including: SNR (the higher the SNR, the more accurately signal attenuation can be measured with higher b-values); echo time (the smaller the b-value, the shorter the achievable echo time); and other factors that are more difficult to assess such as motion artifacts (in general, smaller b-values produce fewer artifacts) [21]. Measurements of diffusion anisotropy tend to be quite sensitive to image noise [22], even though DTI measurement accuracy may be improved by either increasing the number of encoding directions or increasing the number of averages. Unfortunately, this increases the scan time for DTI data collection [23].

The information contained in the diffusion tensor can be 'viewed' through the creation of maps of appropriate diffusion indices derived from DTI data. The orientation of anisotropy vectors can be also coded with specific colors. Generally an RGB (red–green–blue) color map is used to indicate the direction of myelin fiber tracts along the three orthogonal planes. Thus, DT-MRI has excellent potential for applications that require high anatomical specificity. Its excellent ability in anatomic functional WM depiction makes this technique an important and innovative tool in pre- and postoperative management of patients with brain lesions [24].

Water diffusion in tissues is highly sensitive to differences in the microstructural architecture of cellular membranes—increases in the average spacing between membrane layers will increase the apparent diffusivity, whereas smaller spaces will lead to lower apparent diffusivities. This sensitivity makes DTI a powerful method also for detecting microscopic differences in tissue properties. However, the interpretation of changes in the measured diffusion tensor is complex and should be performed with care. In particular, FA is highly sensitive to microstructural changes, but not very specific to the type of changes. DTI has been reported in a broad spectrum of applications, such as in the assessment of WM deformation determined by tumors, in pre-surgical planning (figure 1.10), in Alzheimer's disease (to detect the early phase of disease), in schizophrenia, in focal cortical dysplasia and in multiple sclerosis (for plaque assessment).

1.2.7 Spectroscopy

Magnetic resonance spectroscopy (MRS) is an imaging technique that is able to identify the neurochemical environment in a volume of interest (VOI) [25]. Originally, MRS was developed to determine the chemical and biochemical

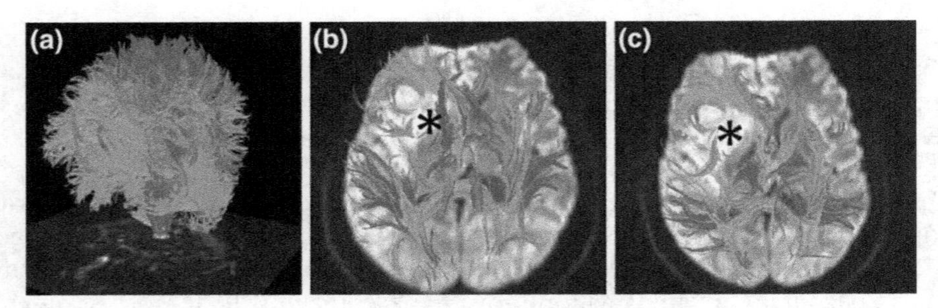

Figure 1.10. (a) 3D reconstruction with fiber tracking from DTI datasets in a patient with right frontal lobe glioma. Axial–oblique view (b) and pure axial view (c), with thin slice segmentation, assessing the relationship between WM fibers and the tumor (*).

properties of some compounds in solution, but with the introduction of gradient field technology its use was extended to *in vivo* studies. ^{1}H, ^{13}C, ^{19}F and ^{31}P represent the isotopes that are more commonly evaluated with MRS in clinical practice.

MRS requires high-intensity static magnetic fields (at least 1.5 T) in order to ensure better homogeneity and increased sensitivity. *In vivo* MR spectroscopy can be performed on the basis of three different parameters: signal intensities, chemical shifts and spin–spin (J) coupling [26]. While the first element provides information on different concentrations of specific compounds, the latter two provide only qualitative assessment on the chemical structure. In particular, the chemical shift considers the resonance frequency difference between the signal of interest (n) and a reference signal (n_{ref}) in relation to the operating frequency of the MR system (n_0). Chemical shifts represent a valid tool in the evaluation of chemical environment properties *in vivo*, since they consider modification in resonance frequencies due to molecular bonding and the distribution of electron density around nuclei.

Resonance signals can be displayed as single peaks (singlets) or can be split into several signals (multiplets). In the final graph of the molecular spectrum, intensities of resonance signals (measured as amplitudes or integrals of the areas under the signals) are proportional to the concentration and to the number of corresponding magnetically equivalent nuclei in a molecule.

Among the various techniques for MRS, the most time-efficient modality is single-voxel spectroscopy (SVS). It analyzes the signal from a specific VOI of a tissue, with a spatial resolution in the range of 1–8 cm^3. Other approaches with multiple voxel sampling, known as chemical shift imaging (CSI) or magnetic resonance spectroscopic imaging (MRSI), can provide metabolite maps. In particular CSI can be extended to cover larger volumes of interest with possible separate voxel-by-voxel analysis; these voxels can be as small as 1 cm^3.

The main limitation of MRS is represented by artifacts due to high differences in magnetic susceptibility (bone, air, large vessels and metals).

The main clinical applications of MRS include the assessment of *N*-acetylaspartate (NAA, d = 2.01 ppm) or creatine (Cr, d = 3.02 ppm). The greater field of application in neuroimaging is represented by oncologic studies. In particular, MRS has been shown to provide further information in terms of the metabolic activity of

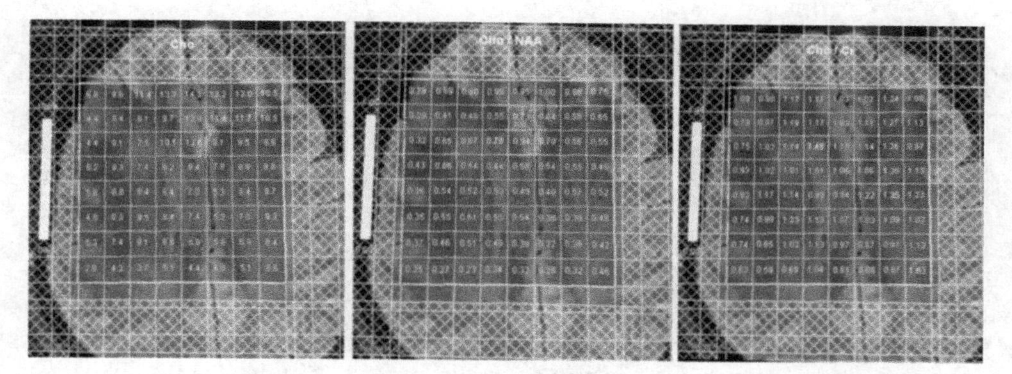

Figure 1.11. Multiple voxel spectroscopy in a patient with solid brain lesions; the images show an assessment of metabolites in the voxels of interest.

neoplastic tissues (figure 1.11). Moreover, its role has recently expanded to the evaluation of painful syndromes, demonstrating a relationship between the concentration of some metabolites in certain brain areas and patient symptoms [27].

In the field of demyelinating diseases, spectroscopy has shown increased choline and lactate levels (indicating the release of membrane phospholipids and the metabolism of inflammatory cells) with decreased NAA levels (indicating neuro-axonal loss or dysfunction) in acute MS lesions. Once the acute phase resolves, there is a progressive return to normal lactate intensities, while choline and lipids show a slower recovery, and NAA levels may remain reduced or show partial recovery for months.

1.2.8 Susceptibility-weighted imaging

Susceptibility-weighted imaging (SWI) is a high-resolution 3D gradient echo technique that is particularly sensitive to the loss of signal intensity created by the disturbance of a homogeneous magnetic field. Various paramagnetic, ferromagnetic or diamagnetic substances, such as air/tissue or air/bone interfaces, can be responsible for these disturbances. In clinical practice, SWI takes advantage of the paramagnetic properties of blood products, allowing an easy identification of intravascular venous deoxygenated blood or extravascular blood products [28]. The intrinsic properties of this new approach make SWI an important tool in the evaluation of several conditions, such as arteriovenous malformations, occult venous disease, multiple sclerosis, trauma and tumors [29].

Sensitivity to susceptibility effects is maximally increased for GE techniques with T2*-weighting, long echo times, and higher field strengths, and is further accentuated through additional post-processing.

Currently, the main application of SWI is the identification of small amounts of hemorrhage/blood product or calcium, which are both possibly unapparent when using other MRI sequences [30].

1.2.9 BOLD functional MRI

Blood oxygenation level-dependent (BOLD) MRI is based on the assumption that a tissue's activity can be estimated by the entity of blood flow in the corresponding volume [31]. Specifically, deoxygenated hemoglobin (dHb) has shown the capability to suppress the fMRI signal generated from neighboring water molecules. The increase in the level of oxygenation of the blood required by the tissue's activity turns into a decrease in dHb suppression, and then into an increase in fMRI signal.

BOLD fMRI can be performed with both SE and GE techniques, with the latter being generally preferred due to their relatively high sensitivity, at the cost of limited spatial resolution. Another protocol, performed with T2*-w sequences, requires administration of iron oxide contrast agents in order to obtain quantitative assessment of blood volume in a determinate tissue. An increase in blood volume to a tissue induces an increase in the content of contrast agents, and consequently a decrease in MRI signal.

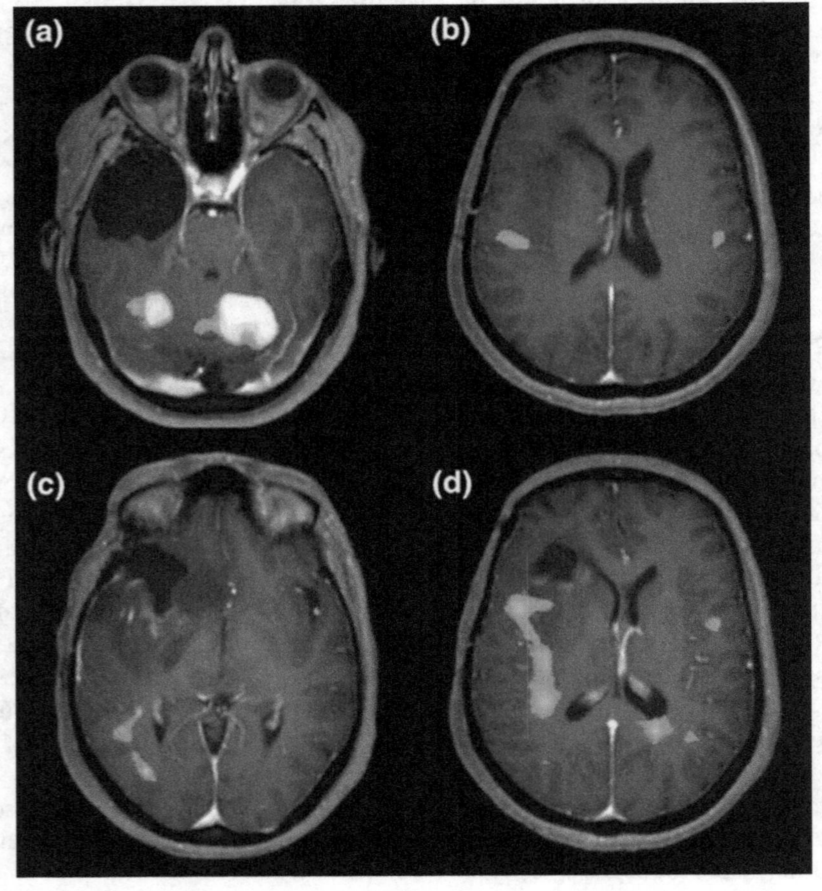

Figure 1.12. Pre-surgical BOLD fMRI study in a patient with a recurrent cerebral tumor. No close proximity was found between the areas of activation (left hand (a),(b) and left foot (c), (d)) and the pathological lesion.

BOLD imaging measures change between alternating states but cannot assess a baseline fMRI signal. Another limitation is represented by the weakness of fMRI signal compared to PET imaging.

However, BOLD fMRI has been shown to represent a valid tool in the clarification of the neural bases of a wide range of sensorimotor and mental processes in neuroscience. For example, initial pain neuroimaging experiences have studied the location and pattern of neural activity evoked by painful or non-painful stimuli. These studies revealed a common whole brain activation pattern (encompassing the primary and secondary somatosensory cortex, cerebellum, anterior insular and cingulate cortices, basal ganglia, and both frontal regions and posterior parietal cortex) responding to mechanical, heat, cold and electrical stimuli, and unique stimuli, referred to as a network or the 'pain matrix' (figure 1.12).

Recent experimental studies have employed BOLD imaging to investigate the mechanisms of cortical reorganization in patients with MS. The results suggest that, at least at some stage of the disease, functional reorganization might play an adaptive role and limit the clinical consequences of disease-related structural damage.

References

[1] Brown M A and Semelka R C 1999 MR imaging abbreviations, definitions, and descriptions: a review *Radiology* **213** 647–62

[2] Lipton M L 2008 *Totally Accessible MRI—A User's Guide to Principles, Technology, and Applications* (Berlin: Springer)

[3] McRobbie D W *et al* 2010 *MRI from Picture to Proton* 2nd edn (Cambridge: Cambridge University Press)

[4] Poustchi-Amin M, Mirowitz S A, Brown J J, McKinstry R C and Li T 2001 Principles and applications of echo-planar imaging: a review for the general radiologist *Radiographics* **21** 767–79

[5] Choyke P L, Dwyer A J and Knopp M V 2003 Functional tumor imaging with dynamic contrast-enhanced magnetic resonance imaging *J. Magn. Reson. Imaging* **17** 509–20

[6] Bali M A *et al* 2011 Tumoral and nontumoral pancreas: correlation between quantitative dynamic contrast-enhanced MR imaging and histopathologic parameters *Radiology* **261** 456–66

[7] Bhooshan N *et al* 2010 Cancerous breast lesions on dynamic contrast-enhanced MR images: computerized characterization for image-based prognostic markers *Radiology* **254** 680–90

[8] Lacerda S and Law M 2009 Magnetic resonance perfusion and permeability imaging in brain tumors *Neuroimaging Clin. N. Am.* **19** 527–57

[9] Meaney J F *et al* 1999 Stepping-table gadolinium-enhanced digital subtraction MR angiography of the aorta and lower extremity arteries: preliminary experience *Radiology* **211** 59–67

[10] Ho K Y *et al* 1999 Peripheral MR angiography *Eur. Radiol.* **9** 1765–74

[11] Wedeen V J *et al* 1985 Projective imaging of pulsatile flow with magnetic resonance *Science* **230** 946–8

[12] Shigematsu Y *et al* 1999 3D TOF turbo MR angiography for intracranial arteries: phantom and clinical studies *J. Magn. Reson. Imaging* **10** 939–44

[13] Walker M F, Souza S P and Domoulin C L 1988 Quantitative flow measurement in phase contrast MR angiography *J. Comput. Assist. Tomogr.* **12** 304–13

[14] Hentsch A *et al* 2003 Gadobutrolenhanced moving-table magnetic resonance angiography in patients with peripheral vascular disease: a prospective, multicentre blinded comparison with digital subtraction angiography *Eur. Radiol.* **13** 2103–14

[15] Luccichenti G *et al* 2003 Magnetic resonance angiography with elliptical ordering and fluoroscopic triggering of the renal arteries *Radiol. Med.* **105** 42–7

[16] Mori S and Barker P B 1999 Diffusion magnetic resonance imaging: its principles and applications *Anat. Rec.* **257** 102–9

[17] Roberts T P and Rowley H A 2003 Diffusion weighted magnetic resonance imaging in stroke *Eur. J. Radiol.* **45** 185–94

[18] Mori S and Zhang J 2006 Principles of diffusion tensor primer imaging and its applications to basic neuroscience research *Neuron* **51** 527–39

[19] Hagmann B P *et al* 2006 Understanding diffusion MR imaging techniques: from scalar diffusion-weighted imaging to diffusion tensor imaging *Radiographics* **26** S205–23

[20] Basser P J, Matiello J and Le Bihan D 1994 MR diffusion tensor spectroscopy and imaging *Biophys. J.* **66** 259–67

[21] Tournier J D, Mori S and Leemans A 2011 Diffusion tensor imaging and beyond *Magn. Reson. Med.* **65** 1532–56

[22] Pierpaoli C and Basser P J 1996 Toward a quantitative assessment of diffusion anisotropy *Magn. Reson. Med.* **36** 893–906

[23] Moseley M E *et al* 1990 Diffusion-weighted MR imaging of anisotropic water diffusion in cat central nervous system *Radiology* **176** 439–46

[24] Pajevic S and Pierpaoli C 1999 Color schemes to represent the orientation of anisotropic tissues from diffusion tensor data: application to white matter fiber tract mapping in the human brain *Magn. Reson. Med.* **42** 526–40

[25] Tran T, Ross B and Lin A 2009 Magnetic resonance spectroscopy in neurological diagnosis *Neurol. Clin.* **27** 21–60

[26] Grachev I D, Fredrickson B E and Apkarian A V 2000 Abnormal brain chemistry in chronic back pain: an *in vivo* proton magnetic resonance spectroscopy study *Pain* **89** 7–18

[27] Kupers R, Danielsen E R, Kehlet H, Christensen R and Thomsen C 2009 Painful tonic heat stimulation induces GABA accumulation in the prefrontal cortex in man *Pain* **142** 89–93

[28] Haacke E M *et al* 2004 Susceptibility weighted imaging (SWI) *Magn. Reson. Med.* **52** 612–8

[29] Sehgal V *et al* 2005 Clinical applications of neuroimaging with susceptibility-weighted imaging *J. Magn. Reson. Imaging* **22** 439–50

[30] Pauling L and Coryell C D 1936 The magnetic properties and structure of hemoglobin, oxyhemoglobin and carbonmonoxyhemoglobin *Proc. Natl. Acad. Sci. USA* **22** 210–6

[31] Vincent K, Moore J, Kennedy S and Tracey I 2008 Blood oxygenation level dependent functional magnetic resonance imaging: current and potential uses in obstetrics and gynaecology *BJOG* **116** 240–6

IOP Publishing

Neurological Disorders and Imaging Physics, Volume 1
Application of multiple sclerosis
Luca Saba and Jasjit S Suri

Chapter 2

Computed tomography principles

Michele Porcu, Antonella Balestrieri, Paolo Garofalo, Jasjit S Suri and Luca Saba

Computed tomography (CT) is one of the radiological techniques most used in clinical practice, and uses x-rays, a type of ionizing radiation. The CT architecture most often used currently is the so called 'third-generation' CT. Spiral multislice-CT allows one to obtain an acquisition that can be reformatted in different ways, in particular using multiplanar reconstruction (MPR), maximum intensity projection (MIP) and volume rendering (VR) techniques. Intravenous contrast medium (ICM) is commonly used in CT in order to better visualize and characterize organs and vascular structures. Dual-energy CT is a relatively recent technique that allows multispectral analysis.

2.1 Basic physics of x-rays

The discovery of x-rays by Wilhelm Röentgen in 1895 opened a new era in medicine. X-rays are highly energetic electromagnetic waves that are able to interact at the atomic level thanks to their short wavelength (between 0.1 and 10 nm). In medical imaging, once the x-rays are emitted they interact with the human body and are then detected by a detection system. The radiological image obtained reflects the interaction of the x-ray beam with different anatomical structures.

Various sources can generate x-rays. In 1913 William David Coolidge invented the so called 'Coolidge tube', which still represents the model based on which modern x-rays tubes are designed, including those used in conventional radiology (CR) and computed tomography (CT). The general principle of a Coolidge tube is very simple [1, 2]: there is a cathode (that consists of a little pigtail wire of tungsten) and an anode (that consist of a plate of tungsten) in a vacuum tube, which are able to generate a spectrum of x-rays according to the potential differences applied to the system (ΔV_1) or the cathode (ΔV_2).

The electrons generated from the cathode by thermionic effects are then accelerated to the anode. The energy released by the impact of electrons on the anode generates heat (99%) and the rest of the energy consists of a spectrum of x-rays, i.e. the 'bremsstrahlung' (produced by the deceleration and deflection of electrons on the crystal structure of the anode) and characteristic x-rays (generated by the interaction of emitted electrons with the electrons of inner orbitals of tungsten atoms) [1, 2].

The intensity of the x-ray beam depends on the number of x-rays emitted from the tube, and it directly depends on the total electronic charge of electrons present on the cathode of the x-ray tube (ΔV_2), according to [1–3]

$$q = t\Delta V_2,$$

where q is the total charge of the cathode and t is time, which in the radiological field is commonly measured in milliamperes per second (mA s).

Further, in accordance with the above, it is important to emphasize that the creation of x-rays is a probabilistic process that does not generate x-rays that are all equivalent to each other, but rather a spectrum of x-rays with different energies and with characteristic peaks of distribution. These features are determined mainly by the material of which the anode is made. The mean energy (E) of the x-ray beam varies according to the total charge of electrons generated by the cathode (q) and the ΔV applied to the tube (ΔV_1), according to [1, 2]

$$E = q\Delta V_1.$$

In the field of radiology, this value of energy is commonly measured in kiloelectronvolts (keV). These parameters can be set to optimize the images produced by the technique and to obtain the best possible ratio between image quality and radiation dose.

The x-rays used in CR and CT can interact with human tissues in different ways, according both to the tissue composition and x-ray spectrum features. These interactions are [1–3] as follows:

- *X-ray scattering* occurs when x-rays are deflected in all directions by the crystalline structure of tissues. This interaction is responsible for the so called scattered effect on the image, also called 'noise'. Increasing the intensity of the x-ray beam tends to reduce the noise of the image and the total ionizing dose (TID) to the patient.
- *The photoelectric effect* occurs when an x-ray hits an electron of the inner orbitals of an atom and gives the electron all of its energy, resulting in ionization of the atom due to the ejection of the electron from its orbital.
- *The Compton effect* occurs when an x-ray hits an electron of the outer orbitals of an atom, giving the electron part of its energy, resulting in ionization of the atom due to the ejection of the electron from its orbital and deflection and loss of energy of the x-ray.

The photoelectric and Compton effects are responsible for the ionizing capability of x-rays, and thus undesirable side effects and non-stochastic (i.e. deterministic) and stochastic (i.e. probabilistic) effects, which need to be considered every time a radiological study is requested/performed.

According to what we discussed previously, when x-rays pass through a patient's body they lose their intensity and reach the detection system, with an intensity (I) smaller than the original (I_0) according to the formula [1–3]

$$I = I_0 e^{-\mu x},$$

where e is the Euler number, μ is the linear attenuation coefficient (specific for every tissue according to its composition) and x is the tissue thickness.

The detection system used in CR was originally a photographic film directly exposed to x-ray beams, whereas it now consists of radiographic cassettes made of photo-stimulable phosphors (to be read by a laser system), or digital x-ray sensors. The images generated in CR are static two-dimensional (2D) images called radiographs, which cannot be used to discriminate the three-dimensional (3D) arrangement of body structures.

CT can be considered an evolution of CR, and it allows one to obtain sectional axial and/or volumetric images of the body, exploiting the same basic principles as CR.

2.2 Introduction to CT

The excellent contrast, spatial and temporal resolutions of modern CT scanners make them essential instruments for the detection and staging of various pathological conditions [3–5]. Contrast resolution is the ability to distinguish two different points on the base of their different intensities, spatial resolution is the ability to distinguish two different points of the image one next to the other and temporal resolution is the time for acquisition of a frame (the shorter the time, the larger the temporal resolution).

CR is still an important instrument in daily clinical practice, in particular as the first level examination for thoracic and orthopedic diseases, but it does not allow a complete and detailed evaluation of deep organs. CT overcomes these limitations, allowing fast evaluation of the structures of the body (in particular with the use of contrast medium), although the radiation doses usually used are higher than in CR. Other techniques such as ultrasonography (US) and magnetic resonance (MR) can be used for the same purposes, and both of these present advantages and limitations when compared to CT. US results are optimal for the first level dynamic examination of vessels and deep organs, and is safer than CT because it does not use ionizing radiation, but the results are inferior to CT because US is operator-dependent and in certain situations, in which air or calcium is interposed between the probe and the organs, its use is impossible. MR, like US, is safer for the patient than CT because it does not use ionizing radiation, and produces better results than CT due to its higher contrast resolution, in particular for the analysis of the central nervous system (CNS). The disadvantages of MR compared to CT lie in the higher execution times of the former (usually more than 20 min) and the inability to perform examinations on patients who suffer from claustrophobia and those with magnetic susceptible metal implants in the body (for example pacemakers or metal fragments).

2.3 CT scanner components

A modern CT scanner consists of a circular gantry, a moving patient table and a control console [3–5]. The circular gantry is made of a solid structure containing an x-ray source and a detection system, which are firmly connected and positioned opposite each other with a 180° angle between them, and a rotation system that rotates the x-ray source and detection system by up to a 360° angle [3–5]. 'Slip-ring' technology, a wireless electrical connection, allows the x-ray source/detection system complex to rotate continuously over 360°, allowing a 'helical scanning' mode (see above) [3–5]. The detection system is connected to a data-acquisition-system (DAS) that converts incidental x-rays into electric pulses, which are in turn managed and analyzed by the computer system in order to create an image series [3–5]. The circular gantry contains a laser sighting system that allows correct positioning of the patient on the moving patient table. The control console allows the radiology technician to control the whole procedure, supported by the radiologist.

2.4 Image acquisition

X-ray beams generated by the rotating x-ray source pass through the patient lying on the moving table in the center of the gantry, and the beams are then detected by the detection system placed opposite the x-ray source. X-rays generated at a known intensity value, equal for every degree of rotation of the system, reach the detection system with an intensity value lower than the initial one. Accordingly, when an x-ray beam generated by the rotating source passes through the human body, it interacts with different kinds of tissues, transferring energy to them. The interaction will depend on tissue composition (water, blood, lipid, bone and crystalline structures) and the rotation degree of the source [3–5].

The detection system is made up of different detectors. Modern CT scanners have solid-state detectors made of rare-earth oxide ceramics, which have high capture and conversion efficiencies (respectively, the capability to absorb x-rays and to accurately convert x-rays in electric signals). The detectors are aligned side by side, divided from each other by thin tungsten septa in order to minimize the detection of scattered radiation, which is responsible for noise in the image. Once the x-ray beams emerging from the human body reach the detection system with intensity value I, they are transformed into electric pulses by the DAS.

These electric pulses are converted into data series and further converted into axial images by the computer, comparing data acquired from acquisitions at different degrees of rotation. The computer represents every scan circle as a matrix (usually a 512×512 matrix) of 3D cubic boxes called voxels [3–5]. Every voxel consists of three mutually perpendicular axes. The z-axis corresponds to the longitudinal axis of the patient, while the x-axis and y-axis are perpendicular to the z-axis.

2.5 Image elaboration

The intensity of the x-ray beam that hits the detection system once it has passed through the human body (I) is correlated to the intensity of the x-ray beam originated by the x-ray source (I_0) according to [1–3]

$$I = I_0 e^{-\int_0^L \mu(x)dx},$$

where e is the Euler number, μ is the linear attenuation coefficient (XLAC) of the x-rays of a specific point of the space, L is the distance covered by the x-ray beam and x is the thickness of the tissue.

According to the following formula, derived from the formula above [3–5],

$$\int_0^L \mu_{(x,y,z)}(x)dx = -\frac{1}{L}\ln\left(\frac{I}{I_0}\right),$$

knowing the values of I, I_0 and L, the DAS is able to calculate the XLAC of every single point of the space, i.e. the XLAC of every single voxel of a pre-set matrix according to the three axes of the space ($\mu_{x,y,z}$). Different algorithms, in particular filtered back-projection (FBR) and iterative algorithms [3–5], are used in CT to calculate the XLAC of every projection obtained during a 180° rotation. The XLAC value is then mathematically converted into a numeric value called the CT number, that corresponds to the density of the tissue included in the voxel, according to the formula [3–5]

$$\text{CT number(HU)} = [1000\ x\ (\mu_{(x,y,z)} - \mu_{\text{water}})]/\mu_{\text{water}},$$

where μ_{water} is the attenuation coefficient of water, μ of air is 0 due to the fact that the x-ray beam is not attenuated along its route and the unit of measurement of the CT number is called the Hounsfield Unit (HU). In the Hounsfield scale the value of water is 0, bone is +1000 and air is −1000; fat shows negative values, whereas blood and abdominal organs show positive HU values [3–5]. This concept is fundamental for the correct interpretation of imaging findings (e.g. a steatosic liver will show HU values lower than a non-pathologic liver because in steatosis liver cells contain more lipids than normal liver cells).

The 3D voxels included in the matrix (usually 512 × 512) are then converted into 2D pixels with a defined CT number using a predefined kernel, an algorithm of reconstruction, and all the axial images are visualized as the observer looks at the patient from the feet (the right side of the image corresponds to the left side of the patient and vice versa) (figure 2.1). There are different algorithms that allow one to obtain 'smoother' or 'sharper' images according to the region analyzed and the radiologists' preferences. Sharp kernels such as B46f are preferred for evaluation of structures such as lung and bone, where tissues differ for very high density values, while smooth kernels such as B20f allow one to evaluate structures such as abdominal and mediastinal organs that differ from one another for lower grades of density [3–5]. According to the CT number, a different shade of gray of a

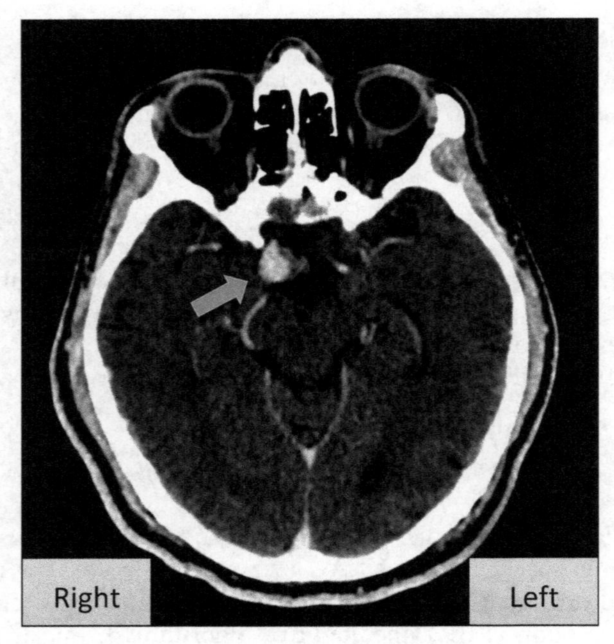

Figure 2.1. Axial image of an ANGIO-CT of the circle of Willis, using contrast medium and a smooth kernel (B20f) executed in order to evaluate an aneurism of the C7 segment of the right internal carotid artery (red arrow). The timing of the CT scanner was set in order to visualize iodinate contrast medium (ICM) inside the arterial vessels (no venous vessels are opacified).

grayscale is assigned to every pixel of the image. Specifically, pixels with higher HU values will tend to be brighter (for example bone), while those with lower HU values will tend to be darker (for example air).

Medical monitors are able to show about 250 shades of gray, although there are 2000 possible values of the Hounsfield scale. Further, the human eye can distinguish about 100 shades of gray, so more HU values will be grouped in a single gray shade. The analysis of radiological images requires selecting the window of view, namely selecting the window center (e.g. 0 HU for water) and the window width (the range of CT numbers to display). This process is called windowing, and it allows one to change the contrast resolution of the image in order to better visualize anatomic details.

The analysis of tissues that differ for very low HU (such as the liver and kidney) requires a window center at 20–40 HU and a narrow window width (400–500 HU) in order to have greater contrast resolution. In the case of bone, a higher window center (550–600 HU) and a larger window width (2000 HU) are necessary [3–5].

2.6 CT generations

Traditionally, five generations of CT scanner have been produced and commercialized [3–5].

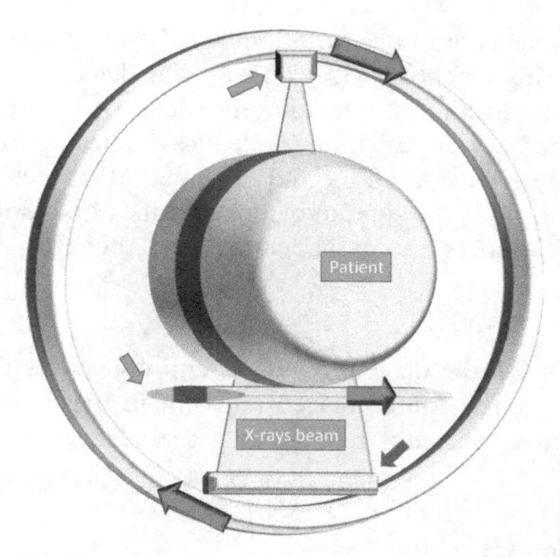

Figure 2.2. A diagram of a third-generation CT scanner. The x-ray beam generated by the x-ray source (green arrow) passes through the patient placed on the moving table (orange arrow) and impacts the detection system (purple arrow). The complex x-ray source and detection system rotates continuously inside the gantry, and the table moves along the *z*-axis.

2.6.1 First-generation CT

The first CT scanner (MARK 1) was introduced in 1972. It was a head scanner consisting of a box-shaped gantry for the patient's head, with an x-ray source generating a very narrow beam and a detection system made of a couple of detectors placed in two adjacent rows. The complex x-ray source–detection system moved into the gantry following a translation–rotation process with an overall 180° rotation. A single axial head scan required an approximately 20 minute scan of the head, with a slice thickness of 13 mm.

2.6.2 Second-generation CT

Second-generation CT differs from first-generation because the x-rays are emitted as a narrow cone-beam and the detection system consists of multiple detectors placed on a single row. The system moves around the patient with translation–rotation movement. The system is also equipped with a moving table, a laser indicator and a gantry tilting system, making the execution of body scans possible for the first time. The scan time is inferior compared to first-generation CT and a scan of a single slice of the chest was possible holding one breath—movement artifacts are thus frequent.

2.6.3 Third-generation CT

This generation of scanners are the most commonly used in current clinical practice. This type of scanner consist of a single x-ray source that generates a wide beam and that is able to interact with a rotating detection system made up of multiple detectors aligned one to each other, originally in a single row (figure 2.2). The system moves according to a simple continuous rotation with 360° movement, thanks to the introduction of slip-ring technology (see above). The detection system is made up of multiple detectors placed on multiple adjacent slices, making it possible to cover a greater section of the body in less time (multislice-CT technology).

Some manufacturers have more recently included other technical solutions, such as fast kV switching x-ray tubes, double x-ray tubes and double-layer detection systems, making multi-energy analysis possible (see above).

2.6.4 Fourth-generation CT

In fourth-generation CT the detection system entirely covers the inner part of the gantry, with a single x-ray source placed adjacent to the detectors rotating in the gantry. This generation has not had great success, mainly because of the high production costs.

2.6.5 Fifth-generation CT

This generation of scanners was designed to scan fast moving organs, in particular the heart. Electron beam computed tomography (EBCT) consists of a cathode from which electrons are accelerated to four semicircular anodes placed around the patient, and diverted by an electromagnetic field, generating an x-ray beam. These types of scanners have not had great success, mainly due to their high cost and technical limitations, despite their high temporal resolution (about 50 ms).

2.7 Spiral volume scanning and multislice-CT

With the introduction of 'slip rings' a new era began in CT [6]. Before this innovation, scanners were only able to perform axial sequential scans (slice-by-slice) due to the presence of electric cables that limited the movement of the x-ray source–detection system.

'Slip-ring' technology allows a continuous rotating movement of the x-ray source and detection system. During the scan, the table moves consensually along the longitudinal axis of the patient (also called the z-axis; the x- and y-axes are perpendicular to the z-axis and represent the coordinates of the axial images).

In the early 1990s, Kalender *et al* developed the algorithm of spiral volume scanning (spiral or helical-CT). This innovation, together with the introduction of multiple rows of detectors aligned in arrays side by side (multislice-CT) [7], allowed faster scans to be obtained and provided the ability to reformat data in order to obtain images on the three planes of the space.

The latest manufacturing developments in CT-scanner technology, such as dual and multi-energy scanners, are described above.

2.8 Post-processing

Currently, every radiological investigation is collected as a digital file called a DICOM (digital imaging and communication in medicine). This can be read and analyzed on personal computers using different software, and most of them are able to reformat images in different ways, thanks to specific algorithms. This action is commonly called the 'post-processing' phase, and it is fundamental for the interpretation of CT scans. The principle post-processing methods used in clinical practice are multiplanar reconstruction (MPR), maximum intensity projection (MIP), minimum intensity projection (MinIP) and volume rendering (VR) [3–7].

MPR is probably the main post-processing method used in clinical practice. It allows users to visualize a CT scan not only in the axial view, but also in the coronal, sagittal and oblique planes. Optimal results are obtained using thin layer reconstructions (maximum 1 mm) (figure 2.3).

MIP allows one to obtain images constituted of a fusion of a group of consecutive images, assigning to every pixel of the image the highest HU value of the pixel of the consecutive images considered. These images allow one to obtain a better definition of tissues with a high linear attenuation coefficient (for example vessels in contrast medium CT) (figure 2.4).

MinIP is analogous to MIP, but in this case the lowest HU value of the packet of images is taken to obtain the final image. This reconstruction method is helpful in order to identify structures or pathology characterized by a low linear attenuation coefficient, such as pulmonary emphysema.

VR allows one to obtain 3D models from 2D images reconstructed with thin layers (usually $\leqslant$1 mm). In this case the pixels of the images are converted into voxels and then into small polyhedrals. It is possible to modify these models, for example changing colors, in order to emphasize different aspects of the image. The images obtained are usually very impressive, and useful for non-radiologist doctors to approach pathologic findings in a simpler way, for example for presurgical planning (figure 2.5).

2.9 Contrast agents

Radiological studies can be performed with or without a contrast medium (also called a contrast agent). These are substances that, because of their composition, enhance the structures in which they diffuse, improving the contrast resolution of the examination.

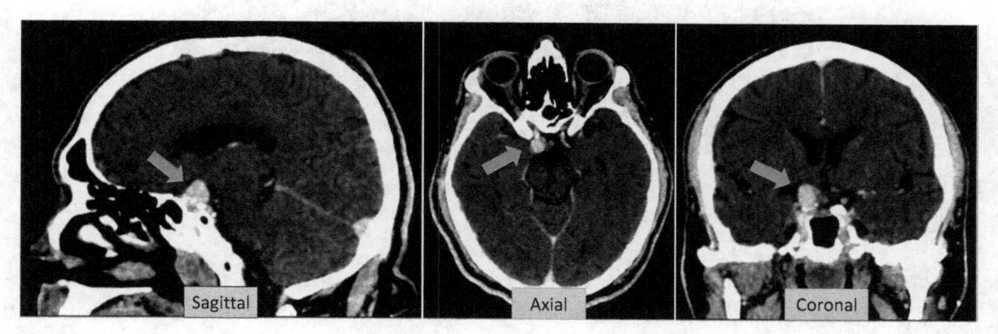

Figure 2.3. MPR reconstructions on the three main planes (sagittal, coronal and axial) of the same case as figure 2.1.

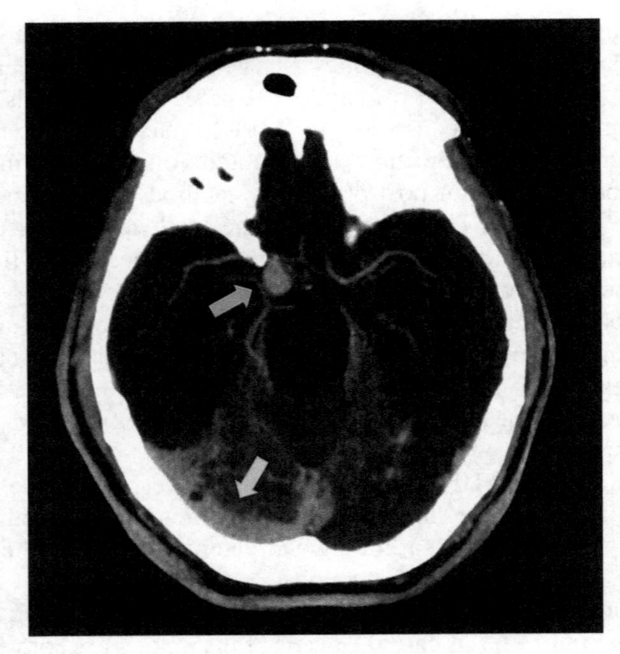

Figure 2.4. MIP reconstruction on the coronal plane of the same case as figure 2.1. It is possible to clearly recognize the aneurism (red arrow); the vessels of the circle of Willis are more recognizable, as well as the right sinus transversus (green arrow).

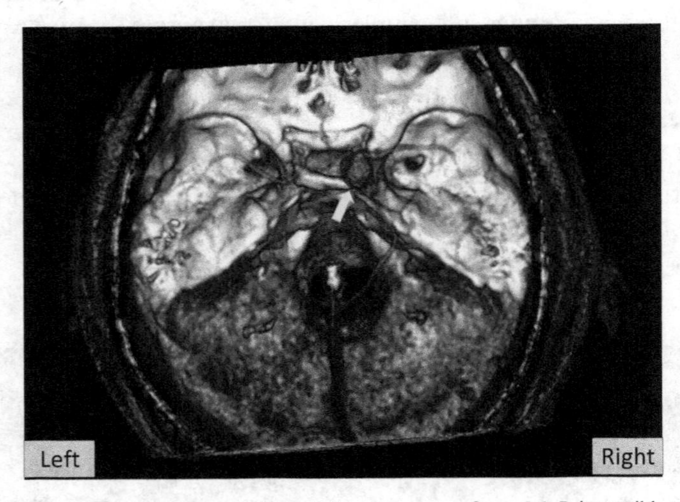

Figure 2.5. VR reconstruction on the coronal plane of the same case as figure 2.1. It is possible to clearly recognize the aneurism (yellow arrow). In this case, the point of view is inverted because the skull is seen from the top.

There are different types of contrast media that can be used in CT:

- *Natural contrast media.* For example, air, water and carbonic dioxide, used in those studies where distension of the GI tract is required, for example CT-enteroclysis or virtual colonoscopy.

- *Non-natural contrast media.* Barium sulfate and diatrizoic acid injective iodinated contrast agents. Diatrizoic acid, as well as air, water and carbon dioxide, are used in CT-enteroclysis in order to make the GI tract opaque. Intravenous iodinated contrast agents are used under various conditions, and are indispensable in certain cases, in particular in vascular CT.

2.10 Intravenous iodinate contrast agents and contrast CT acquisition

Iodinate contrast media (ICMs) are drugs made of organic molecule covalently linked with iodine atoms. The high atomic number of iodine ($Z = 53$) determines its high x-ray linear attenuation coefficient (μ). ICM is injected intravenously, it spreads in the plasma linked to plasmatic proteins, and then to interstitial spaces (there is no intracellular spread) [3, 8].

ICM is filtered and eliminated by the kidney and minimally by the liver. In healthy people, around 85% of the total amount of ICM is eliminated 12 h after administration, and 95% between 24 and 96 h.

These drugs may be divided into [3]:

- *Ionic ICM* (ioxaglate, metrizoate or diatrizoate). These drugs tend to have high osmolality (except ioxaglate) and they are no longer used because of this high osmolality and the consequent high risk of contrast induced nephropathy (CIN).
- *Non-ionic ICM* (iomeprol, iopromide, iopamidol, iohexol, ioxinal and iodixanol). Most non-ionic ICMs are used in clinical practice, at different iodine concentrations (up to 370–400 mg dl^{-1}).

It is important to underline that the parameters of every CT examination (the amount of contrast medium, fluxes, number of scans and scan timing) should be tailored according to the clinical suspect, patient parameters and health conditions, and the ICM and CT scanner used [8].

The examination type is the first parameter to be taken into account. Examinations focused on the study of arterial structures (for example coronary CT angiography, carotid CT angiography) require high fluxes and lower total amounts of ICM, apart from those calculated based on weight. In contrast, examinations that analyze parenchymal and venous structures require higher doses and lower fluxes [8].

Depending on the study, adequate venous access that is able to sustain the required flux needs to be chosen (and, if not possible, the examination needs to be adapted to the venous access obtained). For arterial studies fluxes between 4.0–7.0 ml s^{-1} are required, while for parenchymal studies 2.5 ml s^{-1} could be enough. The total amount of ICM to be administered is calculated on the basis of the patient's weight. Usually parenchymal studies require 1–1.5 ml of ICM per kg of body weight for 320–370 mg dl^{-1} iodine concentration, whereas angiographic studies require smaller amounts because the volume to be studied is smaller. A saline bolus is usually administered following ICM infusion (usually 20–30 ml) in order to compact the ICM bolus and to wash out the venous access in order to both limit adverse reactions in the injection site and avoid beam-hardening artifacts in the arterial phase due to the presence of contrast medium in peripheral veins.

One parameter that is useful in planning CT examinations is the iodine delivery rate (IDR), obtained using

$$\text{IDR [mgI s}^{-1}] = \frac{\text{ICM concentration [mgI ml}^{-1}] \times \text{ICM volume [ml]}}{\text{ICM infusion time [s]}};$$

the higher the IDR, the higher the x-ray attenuation.

It is important to remember that these indications are variable and need to be evaluated and corrected for every single patient, because the optimal amount of contrast medium depends not only on the weight but also on the structure and composition of the body (adipose tissue is less vascularized than other soft tissues, and the vascular structures of tall patients have larger volumes than those of short patients) and the presence/absence of heart failure (reduced heart function could require increased scan times) [8]. Further, other important factors to be taken into consideration are, of course, the CT scanner's technical features, in particular z-axis coverage and resolution time.

Further, we must remember that in several cases dual or multiphase ICM infusion can be used, adopting different flows and/or mixtures of saline solution and ICM.

The evaluation of contrast medium spread in human vessels during its administration, in order to correctly choose the correct time of acquisition of the CT scan, is possible by relying on commonly known physiological circulation times or using one of two more precise methods [3–5]:

- *Bolus tracking*. On the basis of the scanogram (the preliminary scan that allows the limits of the study and the correct field of view to be chosen), the radiology technician can choose a single slice that will be sequentially scanned in order to evaluate the progressive increase of the HU mean value of a determined region of interest (ROI) after ICM infusion. This technique is commonly adopted, for example, to scan and monitor the increasing HU value of the descending aorta and to start the scan once the aorta is opacified to the desired level (for example, when an arterial phase of the whole abdomen is required).
- *Bolus test*. This method is similar to bolus tracking, but in this case a single injection of a small amount of ICM (10–15 ml) is used in order to evaluate the arrival time of the contrast agent in the desired ROI and this is then used to calculate the scanning time.

On the basis of the scan and ICM administration times, ICM will spread in different areas of the body. For example, in the case of CT for suspected pulmonary embolism, a so-called angio-CT scan is required. The CT scan is acquired very soon after IV ICM administration in order to scan the lungs when the greatest amount of ICM will be localized in the pulmonary circle and to find any minus images as suspects for emboli. A subsequent scan of the same district, obtained for example 60–80 s after the beginning of ICM injection, will better enhance mediastinal structures such as nodes.

2.11 ICM: adverse events

Like other drugs, ICMs can cause several adverse reactions, which are important to recognize and manage. Several guidelines have been purposed by different scientific organizations, in particular by the American College of Radiology (*ACR Manual on Contrast Medium*, v10.3) [9] and by the European Society of Urogenital Radiology (*ESUR Guidelines on Contrast Agents*, 10.0) [10]. In this section we will cover the recent recommendations of ESUR [10].

Adverse reactions following intravenous ICM infusion can be divided into:

1. Renal adverse reactions: post-contrast acute kidney injury (PC-AKI).
2. Non-renal adverse reactions: acute and delayed.

PC-AKI is defined as an increase of serum creatinine >0.3 mg dl^{-1}, or >1.5 times baseline, within 48–72 h of intravascular administration of ICM [11, 12]. Known risk factors are: (a) eGFR <30 ml $min^{-1}/1.73\ m^2$ (calculated according to the CKD-EPI formula) before ICM injection or intra-arterial ICM administration with second pass renal exposure and (b) known or suspected acute renal failure [11, 12]. In order to limit the risk of PC-AKI, recent serum creatinine evaluation is required for all patients before ICM intravenous administration, within 7 days in patients with acute disease, deterioration or hospitalization, and within 3 months in all other cases. In those cases in which the execution of an alternative diagnostic examination is not possible, i.e. eGFR measured with the CKD-EPI formula is >30 ml $min^{-1}/1.73\ m^2$, or the patient suffers from severe congestive heart failure (grade III–IV NYHA), adequate hydration with intravenous infusion of 0.9% saline 1 ml $kg^{-1}\ h^{-1}$ for 3–4 h before and 4–6 h after contrast medium is recommended. This same protocol must also be adopted in those emergency cases where the measurement of serum creatinine levels is not available [11, 12]. eGFR 48 h after ICM administration is recommended for at-risk patients, and in the case of PC-AKI diagnosis, regular clinical monitoring and assistance is required. Patients who take metformin with eGFR <30 ml $min^{-1}/1.73\ m^2$ must stop metformin consumption 48 h before contrast medium administration in order to avoid the appearance of lactic acidosis; metformin therapy can be started again 48 h after examination [11, 12].

Non-renal adverse reactions can be divided into acute (those which occur within 1 h from ICM administration) and delayed (after 1 h). Acute non-renal adverse reactions are allergy-like (IgE or non-IgE mediated), hypersensitivity reactions or chemotoxic responses. According to their severity, they can be classified as:

- *Mild reactions* (no medical care required): mild urticaria, mild itching and erythema (grade 1 according to the Ring and Messmer classification), nausea/mild vomiting, warmth/chills, anxiety or vasovagal reactions with spontaneous resolution.
- *Moderate reactions* (medical care required, but not life-threatening): marked urticaria (grade 1 according to the Ring and Messmer classification), mild bronchospasm and facial/laryngeal edema (grade 2 according to the Ring and Messmer classification) and vasovagal reactions.

- *Severe reactions* (life-threatening, management required): hypotensive shock (grade 3 according to the Ring and Messmer classification), respiratory or cardiac arrest (grade 4 according to the Ring and Messmer classification), arrhythmia and convulsions.

The exact frequency of these episodes is not known, partly because many of them are still underreported. Patients at risk of adverse acute non-renal reactions are those with a history of previous moderate or severe acute reaction to an iodine- or gadolinium-based contrast agent, and patients with asthma or atopy that require medical treatment. In the past few years, an anti-allergic premedication protocol base on the use of steroids (prednisone 30 mg or methylprednisone 32 mg, 12 and 2 h before the injection) has been suggested, the new recent ESUR guidelines underline that 'Premedication is not recommended because there is not good evidence of its effectiveness'. Unfortunately, premedication is useful to avoid mild and moderate adverse reactions, whereas it seems to have no effect on severe reactions. In those cases in which an acute severe reaction occurs, the medical and paramedical staff have to act quickly, in particular in those cases in which the patient manifests severe acute adverse reactions, and the location must be equipped with the basic cardiac and advanced life support equipment for the patient. Among the delayed non-renal adverse reactions (that appear 1 h after ICM injection), it is important to remember skin reactions (in particular in patients undergoing treatment with interleukin 2) and thyrotoxicosis.

2.12 Dual-energy CT

The x-rays used in clinical practice in CT are generated with values of ΔV_2 between 70 and 140 kV. For these values, the spectrum of their energy is between 30 and 140 keV, with a mean energy of 56 keV when a ΔV_2 value of 80 kV is adopted, and 76 keV when the ΔV value is 140 kV [13–15].

X-rays interact with molecules of the human body by Compton scattering (when an x-ray hits an electron of the more external orbitals (or shells), which has a low binding energy), or through the photoelectric effect when an x-ray hits an electron of the innermost orbital (known as a K-shell), losing all its energy and knocking the electron out of its orbital. The K-shell binding energy (KBE) is directly related to the atomic number [13–15]. KBE values will be smaller for atoms such as hydrogen ($Z = 1$), carbon ($Z = 6$), nitrogen ($Z = 6$) and oxygen ($Z = 8$), with a mean value between 0.01 keV and 0.53 keV. Calcium ($Z = 20$) and iodine ($Z = 53$) have larger KBE values, 4.0 and 33.2 keV, respectively. The probability of photoelectric interaction is greater when the x-ray energy is similar to the KBE of the electron, and more in general for lower values of ΔV_2 of the x-ray tube. For values of x-ray energy just above the KBE, the x-ray will not reach the detection system since all its energy will be dissipated in the expulsion of the electron from the K-shell, and the relative pixel of the image will show a large HU value [13–15].

This phenomenon is exploited in so-called 'dual-energy' CT. It is possible to characterize the material composition of the tissues by analyzing them with two different x-ray spectra, produced with two different values of ΔV_2, in clinical practice 80 keV and 140 keV because it has been seen that at these values of energy we have the greatest difference and least overlap between the two created spectra. Materials composed of elements with high atomic numbers (calcium and ICM) will show greater variation in the attenuation curves when compared to tissues rich in low-atomic number elements [16, 17].

The use of specific algorithms allows one to create, for example, accurate iodine maps in order to detect areas where ICM tends to accumulate more (for example

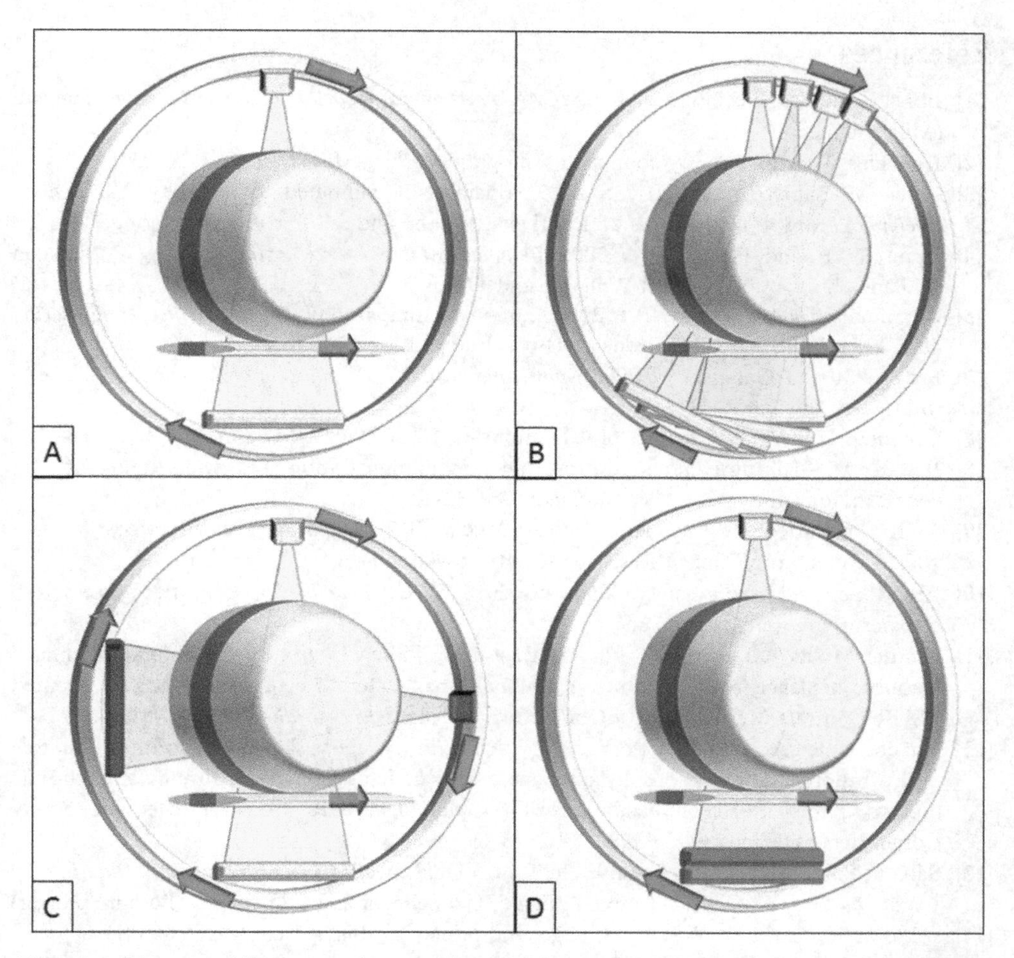

Figure 2.6. Diagrams of CT scanners that are able to exploit the dual-energy technique. (a) A traditional third-generation CT scanner. (b) A fast kV switching tube: the x-ray tube changes the kV and thus the x-ray beam spectrum multiple times during a single rotation (140 kV = yellow triangle; 80 kV = orange triangle). (c) A dual source CT scanner: two different x-ray tubes and two different x-ray detection systems are placed at 90° to one another and rotate at the same time around the patient, using two different kV values (140 kV = yellow triangle; 80 kV = orange triangle). (d) Dual-layer technology: an x-ray beam is emitted by a single x-ray source at 140 kV, and the detection system is composed of an inner layer (green) capable of selectively detecting x-rays with low keV values, and an outer layer (blue) that is able to selectively detect x-rays with high keV values.

vascularized portions of tumoral lesions), or to characterize the composition of kidney stones [16, 17].

The dual-energy technique can be performed on specific CT scanners equipped with a fast kV switching x-ray tube (able to automatically switch the ΔV_2 value of the tube multiple times during a single rotation of the tube), a double x-ray tube (capable of emitting two different x-ray beam at two different ΔV_2 values at the same time) or a dual-layer detection system (able to selectively detect x-rays at higher and lower energies emitted from a single x-ray source at 140 kV) [13–15] (figure 2.6).

References

[1] Borsa F and Scannicchio D 2004 *FISICA Con Applicazioni in Biologia e in Medicina* 2nd edn (Milan: Unicopli)

[2] Kalender W A 2006 X-ray computed tomography *Phys. Med. Biol.* **51** R29–43

[3] Porcu M, Saba L and Suri J S 2015 Principles of computed tomography *3D Imaging Technologies in Atherosclerosis* ed R Trivedi, L Saba and J S Suri (Berlin: Springer)

[4] Brant W E and Helms C A 2006 *Foundamentals of Diagnostic Radiology* 3rd edn (Philadelphia, PA: Lippincott Williams and Wilkins)

[5] Cunningham I A and Judy P F 2000 Computed tomography *The Biomedical Engineering Handbook* 2nd edn ed J D Bronzino (Boca Raton, FL: CRC Press)

[6] Prokop M and Galanski M 2002 *Spiral and Multislice Tomography of the Body* 1st edn (Stuttgart: Thieme)

[7] Goldman L W 2008 Principles of CT: multislice CT *J. Nucl. Med. Technol.* **36** 57–68

[8] Bae K T 2010 Intravenous contrast medium administration and scan timing at CT: considerations and approaches *Radiology* **256** 32–61

[9] ACR Committee on Drugs and Contrast Media 2017 *Manual on Contrast Media* Version 10.3 https://acr.org/Clinical-Resources/Contrast-Manual

[10] ESUR Contrast Media Safety Committee 2018 *ESUR Guidelines on Contrast Agents* v 10.0 http://esur-cm.org/index.php/en/

[11] van der Molen A J *et al* 2018 Post-contrast acute kidney injury. Part 1: definition, clinical features, incidence, role of contrast medium and risk factors: Recommendations for updated ESUR Contrast Medium Safety Committee guidelines *Eur. Radiol.* **28** 2845–55

[12] van der Molen A J *et al* 2018 Post-contrast acute kidney injury. Part 2: risk stratification, role of hydration and other prophylactic measures, patients taking metformin and chronic dialysis patients: Recommendations for updated ESUR Contrast Medium Safety Committee guidelines *Eur. Radiol.* **28** 2856–69

[13] Saba L, Porcu M, Schmidt B and Flohr T 2015 Dual energy CT: basic principles *Dual Energy CT in Oncology* ed C N De Cecco, A Laghi, U J Schoepf and F G Meinel (Berlin: Springer)

[14] Johnson T R 2012 Dual-energy CT: general principles *Am. J. Roentgenol.* **199** S3–8

[15] Flohr T and Schmidt B 2014 Dual energy computed tomography: tissue characterization *Multi-Detector CT Imaging: Abdomen, Pelvis and CAD applications* ed L Saba and J S Suri (London: Taylor and Francis)

[16] Jinzaki M, Yamada Y, Yamada M and Kuribayashi S 2014 Computed tomography multispectral imaging *Multi-Detector CT Imaging: Abdomen, Pelvis and CAD applications* ed L Saba and J S Suri (London: Taylor and Francis)

[17] Simons D, Kachelriess M and Schlemmer H P 2014 Recent developments of dual-energy CT in oncology *Eur. Radiol.* **24** 930–9

IOP Publishing

Neurological Disorders and Imaging Physics, Volume 1
Application of multiple sclerosis
Luca Saba and Jasjit S Suri

Chapter 3

Functional MR applied to neurological disorders

Luigi Barberini

Brain activity, the result of the interaction between brain regions to support all human functions, can be analysed in terms of the networking of single components, neurons, connected at different levels of scale, starting from the single neuron to the size of brain regions, at both the cortical level and in the inner brain structures.

Every action of a person activates a network of connected areas in the brain. Cortical areas and internal structures have been studied with various neurological techniques, such as functional magnetic resonance imaging (fMRI), to encode their functions and activities. Brain biochemical circuits have been identified that are capable of modulating the higher functions, such as movement, memory, behaviour and expression. Through the theory of networks, a mathematical explanation of some of the most incredible properties of the brain can be introduced. fMRI applied to the connection of brain areas (fcMRI), can provide many more answers on the functioning of the human brain in both normal and pathological conditions.

3.1 Network medicine

In many phenomena of the physical world, organisation is not imposed but arises spontaneously from the interactions at the local level of the constituent parts. In this way, short-range interactions generate so-called 'self-organisation' [1]. Populations and markets, and also tissues, organs and systems constituting plants and animals, behave as they were a specific project, but in reality they show properties emerging from below, from the aggregation of individual constituents. The result is a new organisational model that is able to absorb the growing complexity of a context with a strong 'competitive' character [2].

The mechanism is based on four principles:

- *Interconnection* describes the dynamics of the social connection which exploit the so-called small world effect.

doi:10.1088/2053-2563/ab1fdcch3

- *Redundancy* provides for a functional excess of resources whose cost is more than offset in the long term.
- *Sharing* emphasises the importance of a system of common values and functions.
- *Reconfiguration* requires constant adaptation to environmental variations and an ongoing search for new possibilities for devolution.

The concept of emergence from below is a fascinating mystery introduced by this new new science. It could be an interesting future basis for models of human organisations, far from the traditional hierarchical models, allowing free imagination and creativity to build an unpredictable tomorrow. This concept can also open up our understanding of the physical and biophysical sciences, as the evolution of systems is no longer dictated by rigid schemes but by the ability to adapt of the single individual whose final result, however, is 'unpredictable'! These ideas offers an important perspective for the development of 'personalised medicine' that takes into account the genetics of an individual, and also how the system interacts with the environment, i.e. epigenetics. The living cell exchanges energy, matter and information continuously with the surrounding environment. The environment includes the other single cells of the tissue or organ, external stresses such as temperature, biological agents, hunger and satiety, and in general all the states experienced by a living organism depend on the reactions of energy and information exchange with the external environment, at the various levels of aggregation [2]. The chains of reactions that transform one molecule into another by passing through a series of intermediate steps are called metabolic chains, but since cells rarely follow an ordered series in cells, it can happen that various molecules produced downstream of specific chains interact with other molecules previously produced in other chains. This feedback process closes the chain of reactions, and the set of all these processes produces an intricate metabolic network. An organism is, therefore, the result of different stratified networks and is not only the deterministic result of a simple gene sequence. As mentioned, in the new biological models, genomics has been joined by transcriptomics, proteomics and metabolomics. Networks are at the centre of what is called the omic revolution.

Brain activity, the result of the interaction between brain regions to support all human functions, can also be analysed in terms of the networking of single components, neurons, connected at different levels of scale, starting from the single neuron to the size of brain regions, both at the cortical level and in the inner brain structures.

3.2 Brain networks and graph theory

Complex biological systems may be modelled mathematically using graph theory and community detection properties applied to the hub and spoke elements activated in the networking of the fundamental system units.

The human brain operates all functions through connections between different areas, with a set of specific and interacting networks. In the regions of interest, neurons contribute to a locally synchronised activity, and the various regions can work collaboratively with, or are connected to global brain functioning.

External and internal factors may induce functional network alteration. Studies of brain disease can be designed to attempt to identify the self-organisation principles that drive the related functional network alteration.

In this way, it is possible to reveal the properties of the modified system and use these markers for a diagnostic process [3].

Several techniques are available to investigate brain functioning: electroencephalography (EEG), magnetic resonance imaging (MRI) and positron emission tomography (PET). Imaging with magnetic resonance is a crucial tool which is widely used to study brain activity and morphology. Functional MRI (fMRI) is used to investigate how the brain operates different functions. During fMRI, patients can perform particular tasks to highlight the areas of interest activated by the brain to carry out the work (movement tasks, mental calculations, recognition and counting of specific images or sounds transmitted by MRI compatible objects to the patients under examination under controlled and timed conditions).

Recently, the 'resting-state' fMRI approach was developed and applied to explore the modular nature of cortical and subcortical brain functions without task execution by patients. To assess the resting state, functional connectivity (RsFC) seems to be a better investigation method. Functional connectivity is defined as the correlation of the neuronal activity of morphologically separated regions of the brain. In recent years a significant number of studies have started to explore this functional connectivity by measuring this correlation during the resting-state fMRI acquisition of the time series of the blood oxygen level-dependent (BOLD) signal between all the brain regions [4].

Using the well-known calculation environment MATLAB, it is very simple to treat and analyse the time series originated by the time dependence of the BOLD MRI signal. Data can be imported into MATLAB from the usual format used for exchanging files in the imaging sciences, the DICOM format, after transformation of the data into the Analyze format, or the Nifti format. MATLAB [5] is the high-level technical computing language and interactive environment for algorithm development, data visualisation, data analysis and numeric computation used by the members and collaborators of the Wellcome Centre for Human Neuroimaging, directed by Karl Friston, a pioneer in fMRI data analysis [6].

Using the code in MATLAB language, we can read the BOLD signal temporal variation in each voxel of the fMRI experiment and represent the brain time series. A voxel is the small geometric unit used to represent the brain.

The signals represented in figure 3.1 can exhibit a functional correlation introduced by the action of the collaboration of the different brain areas recruited for the task or function.

Using the appropriate coordinates of the voxels, we can read the BOLD signal from each brain region of the fMRI acquisition (figure 3.2).

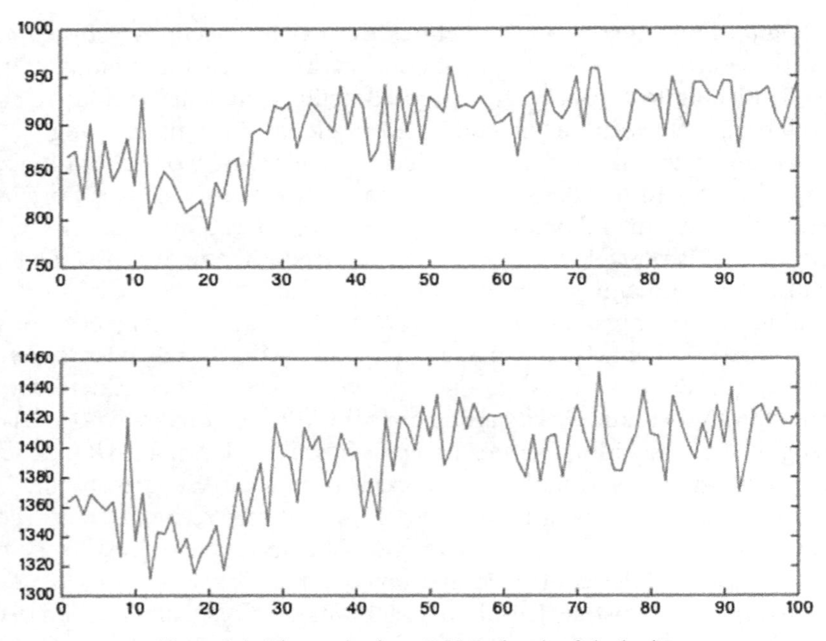

Figure 3.1. Time series from BOLD signals of the brain.

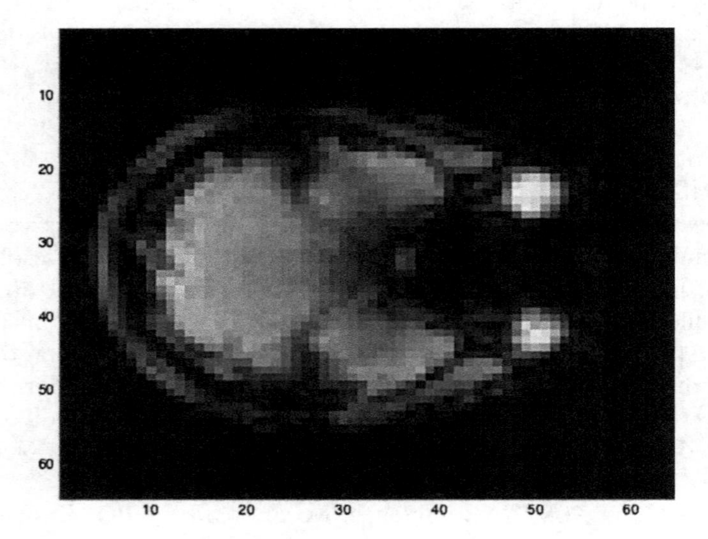

Figure 3.2. fMRI slices brain representation.

In this way, we can study the correlation between each area of the brain during the task or the resting state. Different algorithms extract information about brain activity, and many studies have been produced recently to investigate this activity. The strong correlation between time series can be the basis of the networking between brain areas. These studies have produced a considerable amount of data about networking in the brain and the mechanism of the overall organisation of functional communication in the brain.

However, we can say that one of the most critical applications of fMRI studies is neural activity evaluation and connectivity evaluation in patients with neurological disorders. Neurological disorders usually produce alterations in the functionality of brain regions, but we have to consider the ability of the brain to try to re-establish functional balance by reorganising communication and correlation between the different areas of the brain that can contribute to the execution of the functions.

This behaviour of the brain is defined as 'brain plasticity'; the theory of self-organisation supports the concept of brain plasticity in the complex network [1]. The theory of complexity originated as a result of studies in the field of thermodynamics by the Nobel Prize winner (for chemistry) Ilya Prigogine. Subsequently, the theory was taken up in numerous research centres all over the world, aiming to study complex adaptive systems, i.e. systems characterised by numerous and different elements and by numerous and non-linear connections, which try to adapt their characteristics to maximise the possibilities of evolution. These complex adaptive systems, in order to live and evolve in the environment, self-organise themselves from the inside, without external interventions or pre-established design [1].

Self-organisation is a bottom-up phenomenon, which emerges from the bottom to the top. Hofstadter described, in 1985, self-organisation as 'the spontaneous and unconscious composition of coherent totalities from scattered parts'. Capra, in 2000, emphasised the non-linearity of self-organisation. Even groups of animals and people show similar dynamics, so much so that we often talk about groups that are centred, meaning that the process is not governed by the centre, but by the individual parts of the system [7].

Self-organisation seems to be a prerequisite for the ability to survive or overcome a state of dysfunction, as it generates the types of structures that can benefit from natural and spontaneous action. Only those systems that are spontaneously self-organising may be able to evolve further, and the neurons of various brain structures seem to adapt to operating conditions by modifying the connectivity of functional areas. The brain uses what is self-organised and robust because self-organised features are those that can be modelled more quickly, as reported by Kauffman in 2001 [7].

The most critical variation expected was the circuitry alterations in attention-control brain networks, particularly in syndromes that are borderline between neurological and psychological origins, such as Tourette syndrome. These circuitries, or networks, are related to the cortico-striato–thalamo-cortical circuitry, and fronto-parietal and fronto-striatal networks. We find a different trend in the balance of the 'segregation' (a general decrease in correlation strength) between regions close in anatomical space and 'integration' (an increased correlation strength) between selected regions distant in space.

Neurological disorder categorisation relates [8] to the primary location affected, the primary type of dysfunction involved or the primary type of cause. The broadest division is between central nervous system disorders and peripheral nervous system disorders. Neurological disorders can affect an entire neurological pathway or a single neuron. Even a small disturbance to a neuron's structural pathway can result in dysfunction.

According to the University of California, San Francisco, there are more than 600 different neurological disorders that strike millions each year. These diseases and disorders inflict great pain and suffering on millions of patients and their families, and cost the US economy billions of dollars annually. Social Security approves disability benefits for severe cases of epilepsy, cerebral palsy, Parkinson's disease, multiple sclerosis, ALS and other nerve-based diseases.

Several studies of neurological diseases put the emphasis, in some pathologies, on the role of the cortical-striatal-thalamo-cortical circuits, particularly the subcortical component (such as the basal ganglia) and the cortical component (such as the prefrontal cortex). Neurological disorder populations frequently report atypical brain connectivity correlated to changes in behaviour, motor skills and cognitive abilities. The neural correlates underlying the development of these changes are frequently poorly understood. In particular, we are interested in the involvement of the different system networks that are responsible for self-regulatory control of these abilities.

Modern neurological studies provide an exploration of all the changes in the circuitry of the brain, starting from the 'default mode network' (DMN) activated during the rest state of the brain or specific networks activated during task execution. We mention the pioneering works of Biswal, Lerner *et al*, Wang *et al* and Church *et al* [9–12, 20].

The DMN is defined as the network of brain regions that are active during the awake period but in a rest condition. The DMN is the system of connection between some anatomically defined brain region that is mostly activated when individuals focus on tasks or functions without interacting with external stimuli, such as daydreaming, envisioning the future and retrieving memories. The DMN is active when a person is not focused on the outside world. The DMN has a negative correlation with the brain activity of systems that focus, for example, on external visual and auditory signals. The DMN is one of the most studied networks active during the resting state and is one of the most easily visualised networks, but it is not the only one. There are several other resting-state networks. Functional connectivity studies reveal that some neural networks are strongly functionally connected during rest. The key networks are also referred to as components, and those frequently reported include the DMN, the sensory/motor component, the executive control component, up to three different visual components, two lateralized frontal/parietal components, the auditory component and the temporal/parietal component. As already reported, these resting-state networks consist of anatomically separated but functionally connected regions displaying a high level of correlated BOLD signal activity. These networks are found to be entirely consistent across studies, despite differences in the data acquisition and analysis techniques. It is important to note that most of these components that are active in the rest state represent known functional networks, i.e. regions that are known to share and collaborate with some cognitive functions.

Important aspects of these approaches are the reliability and the reproducibility. Resting-state functional magnetic resonance imaging (RS-fMRI) can visualise the low-frequency fluctuations in spontaneous brain activities, representing a tool for the characterisation of functional connectivity at a macroscopic scale [6]. It is also useful to characterise inter-individual differences in normal brain function and various brain disorders. RS-fcMRI studies suggest reliability and reproducibility for measurements derived from MRI and commonly used in the analysis of functional networks of the human brain. These metrics have great potential to accelerate the identification of early biomarkers for various brain diseases.

3.3 fcMRI and neurological disorders

One of the most recently studied neurological problems is the alteration of the executive functions of attention. Executive functions are those skills that come into play in situations and tasks where the use of routine behaviours and skills is no longer sufficient for success. These are the essential functions of planning and creating strategies. More generally, those cognitive processes are at the basis of problem-solving.

The brain areas involved in attentional executive functions include the fronto-striatal and fronto-parietal systems. The former is responsible for 'self-regulatory control', i.e. self-monitoring cognitive, affective and motor function, the latter is considered responsible for the so-called 'adaptive control' that allows an adjustment in the transition from one event to another.

It is essential to study the relationship between disease and possibly altered whole brain topology. Several experimental approaches have combined studies of neuro-physio-psychological assessment and graph theoretical network analysis of fMRI for particular disorders, such as Tourette syndrome.

In the design of the experiment, it was postulated that, in order to reveal the neural mechanisms that govern tic generation in Tourette syndrome, a motion task, with a higher cost function related to the higher attention requested by difficult motion, should be submitted to patients and healthy subjects to examine neural activity and connectivity within cortico-striatal–thalamo-cortical circuits. Neuroimaging studies have shown that attention (to motion in this case) tasks can increase the responsiveness of several cortical areas, not only the motion-selective ones. An increase or decrease in the activation of a cortical area is often attributed to attentional modulation of the cortical projections to that area. This fact leads to the idea that, in Tourette patients, attention is associated with changes in brain connectivity. The attentional modulation of functional connectivity was addressed using a complex task.

Subjects completed a modified finger tapping motor task, with both the right and left hand, with switching on demand between two conditions: usual finger tapping and finger tapping without the opposition between the thumbs and middle fingers. Subjects were not required to perform the task as quickly as possible. Participants completed a brief practice, running the task before scanning to familiarise themselves with the stimuli and the task requirements. The vocal command to switch between the two conditions was given randomly to increase the difficulty of the task.

All subjects were scanned under identical stimulus conditions. The hypothesis was that the hemodynamic responses addressed by an attentional component of the task can reveal a cortico-striatal–thalamo-cortical network alteration.

3.4 fMRI as an innovative and powerful tool for the investigation of neurological disorders using network medicine

fMRI is a specific MRI technique that indirectly measures brain activity through the effects generated by associated changes in the blood flow of the brain regions operating a task or a function. More specifically, brain activity is measured through oscillation in the frequency of the BOLD signal in the brain.

The technique is the same as classical MRI but uses a fast reading of the voxel activity by using an impulse sequence that can reveal the change in magnetisation between oxygen-rich and oxygen-poor blood measures. Noisy signals frequently corrupt the fMRI experiment, originating from several sources. A statistical approach is used to extract the underlying signal. The resulting brain activation is graphically represented using colour coding maps to represent the strength of activation of the brain region studied. This technique can localise activity into small volumes to within sub-millimetres cubes and, using particular data filtering techniques, a wide temporal range can be achieved.

fMRI is used both in research and in clinical settings to investigate cognitive functions, motor ability, external perception, behaviour, etc. It can also be applied simultaneously with other measures of brain physiology such as EEG.

fMRI can be used for assessing resting brain functions or task-related brain functions. Beginning in the 18th century, physicians began to be aware that a stroke or other brain injury could critically compromise cognitive functions. At that time, the anatomopathologist J Gall proposed that in the brain there were several 'organs', or parts of the brain, responsible for the perception and elaboration of colours, sounds and flavours, and parts of the brain with the task of memorising events, parts of the brain dedicated to speech, as well as parts that characterise behaviours such as friendship, benevolence, pride, etc.

Later, several physiologists tried to verify Gall's theory, but they could find no evidence of the existence of the organs postulated by Gall. For this reason, they claimed that the brain was an undifferentiated and homogeneous unit that generates thought; they said: 'the brain secretes the thought as the liver secretes the bile'.

This concept dominated until the Broca studies of 1860. In autopsies of patients with aphasia, Broca reported damage to the frontal lobe on the left side of the brain. After identifying what is now called the Broca area, he declared: 'we speak with the left hemisphere'. Since then, neurologists have identified different centres responsible for the different activities of the brain, but they have also discovered that these centres rarely work in isolation. The integration, or correlation, of different areas of the brain is crucial to its functioning, and this fact leads to the concept of 'networking'. The networks thus provide a point of conjunction between the paradigm of a brain divided into specific sectors and what it represents as a single entity. The brain consists of different parts in which various structures provide integration between specialised areas. In the cerebellum, for example, the neurons form modules that are repeated several times and the interaction between the various modules is restricted to first neighbours, as happens in other areas of the brain, where we find random connections with a lower probability of connecting local intermediate neurons or distant neurons in the cortex region. Many of the higher functions of mammals combine local structures with more casual long-range connections. Some neuroscientists believe that these connection patterns may be responsible for subjective awareness—the emergence of consciousness may be the result of a sufficiently 'complex' network structure. Identifying the detailed structure of these neuronal networks is extremely difficult, because of the enormous number of cells and the difficulty of acquiring data. When human beings perform a simple action, many electrochemical signals are activated, which cross each neuron through different areas of the brain. These regions can be identified through techniques such as fMRI. Through this technique, it has been discovered that different areas of the brain emit correlated signals. That is, different areas of the brain show a special synchronisation, or correlation, that suggests they can influence each other. These areas are nodes of the network that are connected if there is sufficient correlation. Also at this level, the brain appears as a set of connected elements. Every action of a person activates a network of connected areas in the brain. Many modern studies report attempts to identify similar areas that can be associated with different functionalities. Cortical areas and internal structures have been studied with various neurological techniques to encode their functions and activities. Brain biochemical circuits have been identified as being capable of modulating the higher functions, such as movement, memory, behaviour and expression.

3.5 Physiological basis of fMRI

The physiological blood-flow response, with the BOLD oscillations, has a characteristic temporal range. The primary time resolution parameter used in the sequence is the repetition time, or TR, which indicates how frequently a particular brain slice is excited by MRI pulses and allowed to lose its magnetisation. The values of TR could vary from short times = 500 ms to long times = 3 s. For fMRI specifically, the hemodynamic response is assumed to last over 10 s, rising (that is, as a proportion of current value) with a peak at 4–6 s, and then falling. Changes in the blood-flow system integrate responses to neuronal activity over time. This response is a smooth continuous function, sampled best with a fast TR. This fact helps to map faster fluctuations such as respiratory and heart rate signals and to improve the quality of the information reported.

fMRI measures the neuronal activity in the brain, and other physiological factors can influence the BOLD signal oscillation. For example, respiratory fluctuations and cardiovascular activity influence the BOLD signal measured in the brain, therefore these effects are usually extrapolated and removed during the preprocessing of the fMRI data. For these reasons, many experts approaching the idea of resting-state fMRI were sceptical, and it has only been recently that they became confident that the signal measured is not only an artefact produced by other physiological functions.

Resting-state functional connectivity MRI between spatially distinct brain regions reflects the history of activation and co-activation patterns within these regions and between these regions, thereby serving as a measure of brain plasticity.

fMRI data can be acquired from individuals suffering from neurological pathologies during resting-state acquisition or during task execution on demand between two different conditions. These two different conditions of the task require attention, strategy and strength of maintenance, which are crucial in several brain disorders, including neurodegenerative disorders with motor ability impairments.

As in EEG analysis, it is possible to investigate the BOLD signal using a band subdivision of the BOLD signal frequency range. Using a bandpass filter applied to the time series, we can investigate the potential frequency-modulation of fcMRI measures related to differential actions of brain circuitries in the resting state, for example, motor task control cognitive testing in a Tourette population [13]. Further information on this subject can be found in [14].

A usual fMRI experiment can be performed using a 1.5 T scanner and using a gradient echo-planar imaging sequence for the functional time series acquisition. The fMRI data can be acquired using pre-settled sequences with different names depending on the manufacturer, but typical values for the repetition time and echo time are TR/TE 3000/50, with a flip angle of 90° and a DFOV of 22.8 cm × 22.8 cm on a matrix of 128 × 128.

Robust statistical analysis must address the issue of noise source determination and cancellation in fMRI to avoid possible confounding factors due to, for example, physiological noise. There are many types of software and freeware to analyse fMRI connection data. Using, for example, the functional connectivity toolbox CONN (www.nitrc.org/projects/conn), the software implements the component-based noise correction (CompCor) algorithm for physiological and other noise source reduction strategies. These include the removal of movement and temporal covariates, and temporal filtering of the BOLD oscillations. The noise reduction strategy in CONN does not rely on global signal regression, and it allows for physiological interpretation of anticorrelations.

The spatial preprocessing procedures adopted include slice-timing correction, realignment, coregistration, normalisation and spatial smoothing. The toolbox employs segmentation of grey matter, white matter and cerebrospinal fluid areas for optional use during removal of temporal confounding factors. Spatial preprocessing is implemented in CONN using SPM (Wellcome Department of Imaging Neuroscience, London, UK, www.fil.ion.ucl.ac.uk/spm). SPM and CONN both run under MATLAB (The MathWorks, Natick, MA).

Statistical parametric mapping is carried out in the framework of the general linear model (GLM) [6] (FMRIB Software Library v5.0 by the Analysis Group, FMRIB, Oxford, UK) [15].

3.6 Data-driven analysis, resting state and task methods

3.6.1 Data-driven activation

Clinical, or other kinds of data, can be used to drive the analysis of the time series extracted from the brain activity, both in the resting state or in task-related BOLD signal oscillation. Generally speaking, an index such as the 'Yale-Brown Obsessive Compulsive Scale' (YBOCS), the 'Yale Global Tic Severity Scale' (YGTSS) and the Mini-Mental State (MMSE) test can be used to assess motor, vocal, or other psychological and physiological aspects of brain functioning or cognitive symptom severity in a patient group. Healthy comparison subjects must be accurately selected to match the personal data, and the patient must be excluded if they report any history of different illnesses, in order to reduce the 'noisy information' reported in the analysis. A history of substance use disorder, neurological illness, head injury with loss of consciousness, a medical condition that could affect cognitive functioning, or factors contraindicating fMRI also serve as exclusionary criteria.

3.6.2 Resting-state activation

Resting-state fMRI is used in brain mapping for regional interaction evaluation. These interactions occur in the resting state of the brain, when a specific task is not being performed, or the task-related state.

Some resting-state conditions are identified in the brain, one of which is the DMN (discussed above). These resting-state conditions of the brain generate changes in blood flow in the brain. It creates what is referred to as a blood oxygen level dependent (BOLD) signal. Since brain activity is inherently present even in the absence of a task or external stress, any brain region will have natural variations and fluctuations in the BOLD signal. The resting-state approach is useful for exploring the minimal or basic functional organisation of the brain and for examining whether the functional organisation is altered in neurological disorders.

Research on functional connectivity in the resting state has revealed that some networks are always present in healthy subjects. These networks may represent the different stages of consciousness, and the difference in intelligence found between various animal species may be based on specific patterns of synchronous activity of neurons or functional clusters of neurons.

3.6.3 Task-related activation

An example of a mixed designed strategy is represented by a motor task based on vocal commands (events) given to patients with a block strategy (figures 3.3 and 3.4).

The hypothesis of altered functioning of the network responsible for programming motor function in response to a stimulus (the frontal–parietal network responsible for executive functions) may be the best explanation of the clinical manifestations associated with TS.

A random effects analysis generates one contrast image per individual for the 'switch motion' task. To capture, as well as possible, the effects of interest strictly

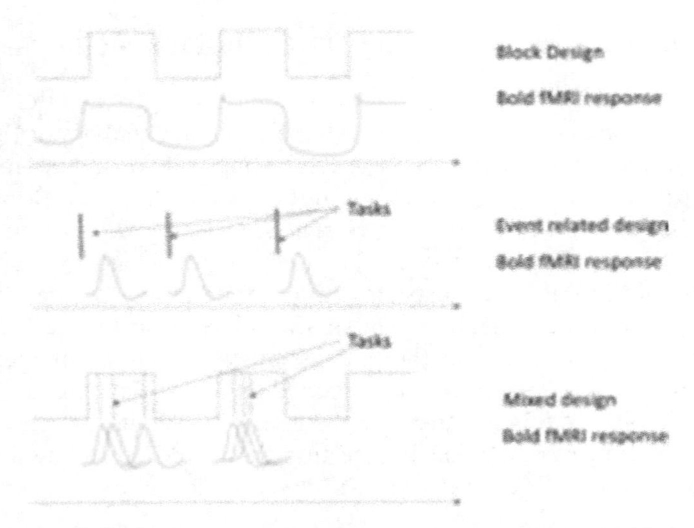

Figure 3.3. Different presentation strategies of the stimulus in a fMRI experiment: (A) block design, (B) event-related design and (C) mixed design [16].

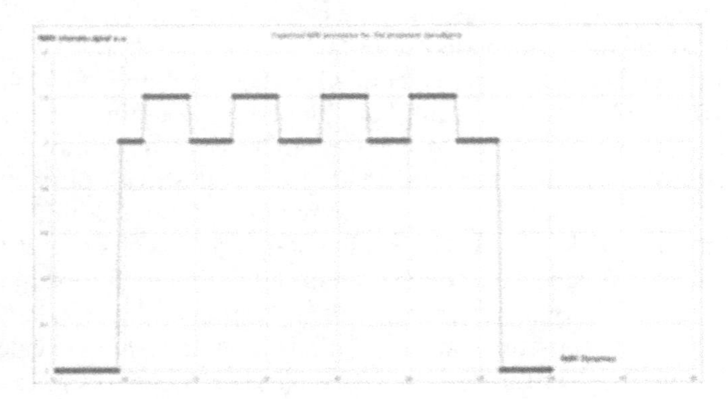

Figure 3.4. Example of a mixed design of fMRI.

correlated to the switching in the motor task (motor strategy organisation) it is analysed as a temporal range of only three dynamics after the vocal command submission. In this way, we aim to produce contrast maps for the fMRI signal and connectivity contrasts for the phoneme of interest. Coordinates of significant activations are expressed in Talairach space.

The location of the local maxima and the associated function are investigated using XJVIEW and Sleuth2.0 (http://brainmap.org) software. The relationships between Tourette syndrome symptom severity, as measured using the YBOCS total score, and brain activation during response inhibition are evaluated.

Due to the expected weakness of the signals, we use a statistical threshold of $p < 0.05$ (uncorrected) for the single subject fMRI activation and a minimum cluster extension of five contiguous voxels to improve the significance of the results [17].

Finally, participant characteristic and behavioural data are analysed using the MATLAB ‘Statistics’ toolbox.

3.7 Connectivity evaluation in the fMRI experiment: from functional MR to functional connectivity MR

Above, we mentioned CONN software as a practical and intuitive tool to perform a network analysis of fcMRI experiments.

From the mathematical point of view, connectivity measures in CONN are performed mainly at the ‘voxel-to-voxel’ level. To discuss the properties of connectivity related to the brain functions that are spatially segregated in the brain, a ‘seed-to-voxel’ and ‘ROI-to-ROI’ analysis can be carried out as a spatial extension of the areas of interest. Brain areas of interest can be spatially labelled using the Brodmann area (BA) codification in order characterise the source regions for the extraction of the time series of interest. The same areas are subsequently used as labels for the targets in the ROI-to-ROI and seed-to-voxel analysis. Usually, the data presented focus on the zero-lagged bivariate-correlation linear measure of functional connectivity between two sources, defined as

$$r = (x^t \cdot x)^{\frac{1}{2}} \cdot b \cdot (y^t \cdot y)^{-\frac{1}{2}}$$

bivariate correlation, where

$$b = \frac{x^t \cdot y}{x^t \cdot x}$$

is a bivariate regression.

This parameter is the voxel-level functional connectivity MRI measure derived from the voxel-to-voxel connectivity matrix $r(x,y)$. In our experiment, we characterise the intensity of the global connectivity parameter between each voxel and the rest of the brain. This calculation is based on the intrinsic connectivity contrast (ICC) measure [18]:

$$\text{ICC} = \frac{1}{|\Omega|} \sum_{y=\Omega} |r(x, y)|^2 .$$

Finally, the graph measure at the ROI and the network level performed are defined as the cost function, expressed at the ROI-level with the measure

$$C_n(G) = \frac{1}{|G| - 1} \cdot |G_n| .$$

The cost function expressed at the network level is the measure

$$C(G) = \frac{1}{|G|} \cdot \sum_{n \in G} C_n(G),$$

where the $C_n(G)$ parameter represents the cost in graph G, and $|G|$ represents the number of nodes in graph G.

3.8 Brain alterations in the Tourette study

Based on this metric, the results for the Tourette syndrome study, obtained with a [0,1:1] Hz bandpass filter and using only the first three dynamics acquired at the switch request, show important features. In terms of the graph theory, an important finding of our study shows that Tourette syndrome altered the global properties of the brain network. It also caused local changes, affecting some important ROIs (figures 3.5 and 3.6). In particular, we find a significant global difference for the cost parameter. Observing the measure for the BA(11) region (tables 3.1 and 3.2):

Cost (p-value uncorrected = 0.05) for the healthy population = 0.96
for the TS population = 0.17.

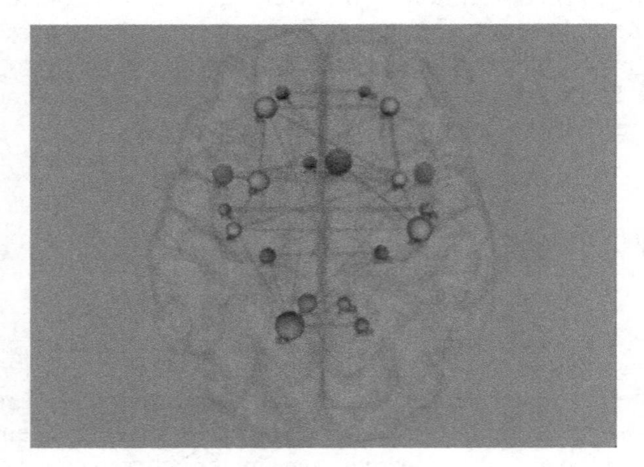

Figure 3.5.

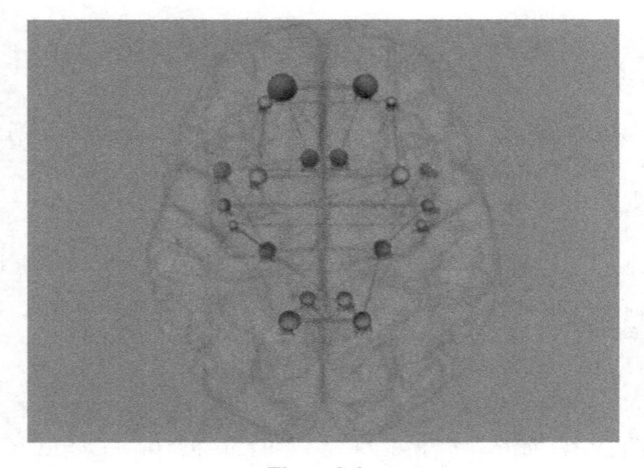

Figure 3.6.

Table 3.1. Network parameters measurements for pathological sample.

BA.11 (*R*). Orbitofrontal cortex						
Global efficiency	Local efficiency	Betweenness centrality	Cost	Average path length	Clustering coefficient	Degree
0.225 685 454 5	0.388 888 833 3	0.036 407 818 2	0.095 694	2.704 403 555 6	0.361 111 166 7	1.818 18

Table 3.2. Network parameters measurements for sample control.

BA.11 (*R*). Orbitofrontal cortex						
Global efficiency	Local efficiency	Betweenness centrality	Cost	Average path length	Clustering coefficient	Degree
0.368 453 555 6	0.639 364 933 3	0.058 068	0.169 591	2.940 627 888 9	0.572 381	3.2222

For the others parameters reported (p-unc = p-value uncorrected):

- Global efficiency (p-unc = 0.05, min 0.23, max 0.37).
- Local efficiency (p-unc = 0.05, min 0.39, max 0.64).
- Betweenness centrality (p-unc = 0.05, min 0.036, max 0.058).
- Average path length (p-unc = 0.05, min 2.7, max 2.9).
- Clustering coefficient (p-unc = 0.05, min 0.36, max 0.57).
- Degree (p-unc = 0.05, min 1.8, max 3.2).

As reported in manuals, Brodmann area 11 is involved in decision making, processing rewards, planning, encoding new information into long-term memory and reasoning.

For the others regions involved, we find as follows: lateral inferior prefrontal cortex right (Brodmann area 44/45), medial frontal gyrus (Brodmann area 46), dorsolateral prefrontal cortex (Brodmann area 9/46), lenticular nucleus (i.e. pallido and putamen) and thalamus.

These regions represent part of the fronto-striatal system. The fronto-striatal system is implicated in the control and inhibition of movements and behaviours. Fronto-striatal circuits are neural pathways that connect frontal lobe regions with the basal ganglia (striatum) that mediate motor, cognitive and behavioural functions within the brain. They receive inputs from dopaminergic, serotonergic, noradrenergic and cholinergic cell groups that modulate information processing. All these findings are critical information for the description of Tourette syndrome. All the results and information originated in 'network medicine'.

3.9 Brain alterations in HIV–HCV patients

Another important application for fcMRI is studies seeking to understand the interactions between non-neurological pathologies and their neuropsychological expression [21]. We report as an example a study carried out for HIV and HCV co-infection using an fMRI and fcMRI approach [22–24]. This study will lead to the development of better models for the pathogenesis of HIV and HCV [19, 25].

According to the known usefulness of RS-fcMRI in assessing abnormalities in neuropsychological testing, the work showed connectivity differences between HIV+ and HIV–HCV groups with equal cognitive performance. The HCV-related modifications of HIV seropositive brain networks identified by our study suggest a synergic effect between HCV–HIV co-infection, with particular involvement of the cerebellum, probably mediated by increased SNC inflammation, and the fronto-striatal system (figure 3.7). Again, such brain systems, which receive inputs from dopaminergic, serotonergic, noradrenergic and cholinergic cell groups, modulate important processes such as information processing [23–25].

Further studies are necessary to confirm the role of RS-fcMRI and if this approach could play a role in identifying patients that can have more cognitive improvement with current HCV therapeutic options [22]. It is important to underline that these are preliminary data, even if the statistical association is robust and further studies to confirm our findings are necessary.

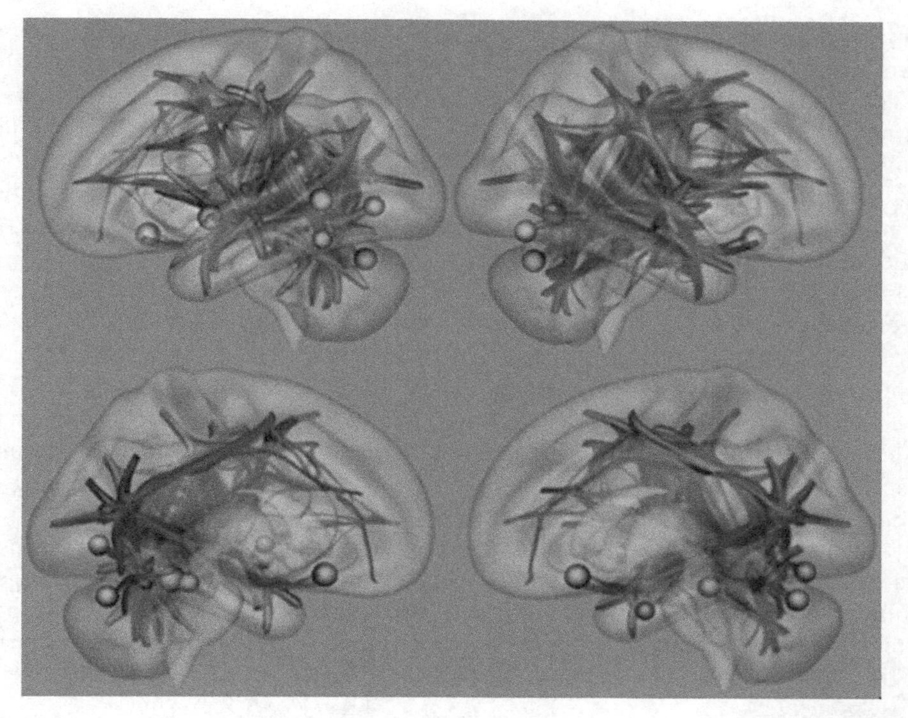

Figure 3.7. Representation of the nodes exhibiting an alteration in the betweenness centrality in the HIV (top) and HIV + HCV (bottom) populations.

3.10 Brain alterations in gustatory stimulus processing

Finally, as an example, we report an interesting fMRI study on the brain default mode network (DMN) alteration induced by the bitter gustatory stimulus. Processing of the gustatory stimulus is altered in several neurological pathologies such as ASD and Parkinson disease [26].

Basically, despite the exhaustive information concerning the role of the physiological structures involved in gustatory stimuli, there is still a need to clarify as to whether the gustatory sense is processed in the human brain and how different stimuli affect the brain areas involved in taste processing. This fMRI study investigated two populations characterised by their opposite response (sensitive/non-sensitive) to bitter gustatory stimulus induced by the propylthiouracil molecule (PROP). In the MRI setting PROP was delivered to the subjects using impregnated filter paper disks. The individuals recruited for this study were three super-tasters and three non-tasters of the bitter stimulus.

Functional data were processed with the toolbox in [6], and network pathways were analysed using the CONN toolbox [15]. The general linear model (GLM) technique was applied allowing for statistical evaluation of activation. Low oscillations of BOLD signal [0.09:0.9 Hz] time series were processed calculating the semi-partial correlation index between voxels. The integrated connectivity contrast measure was applied for connectivity map calculation. All contrasts were examined with a voxel-wise *t*-test ($p < 0.05$ uncorrected).

The study examined activations using the four brain default mode networks, defined by Fox *et al* as crucial seeds for connectivity analysis. A dissimilarity contrast matrix is constructed between the non-taster and super-taster subjects (between the subjects' contrast) and between the two conditions of stimulus submission and no stimulus submission. DMN ROI projections towards the Brodmann areas were detected with the *t*-test significance test.

In this fMRI study the insula, cingulate cortex, somatosensory associative cortex, entorhinal cortex and premotor cortex are more correlated to the four DMN areas during the bitter stimulus processing in the super-taster than in the control population (figures 3.8–3.11).

The study shows that bitter taste is differently processed by the two groups, super-tasters and non-tasters, and suggests further tests to encompass the primary gustatory pathways and their correlations and differentiation in processing and interpreting gustatory information.

It seems likely that further studies are needed to address the possible reasons for this difference between these populations. A working hypothesis can privilege an evolutionary differentiation between these two populations, as the correct appreciation of bitter taste can be an advantageous step in identifying possible dangerous

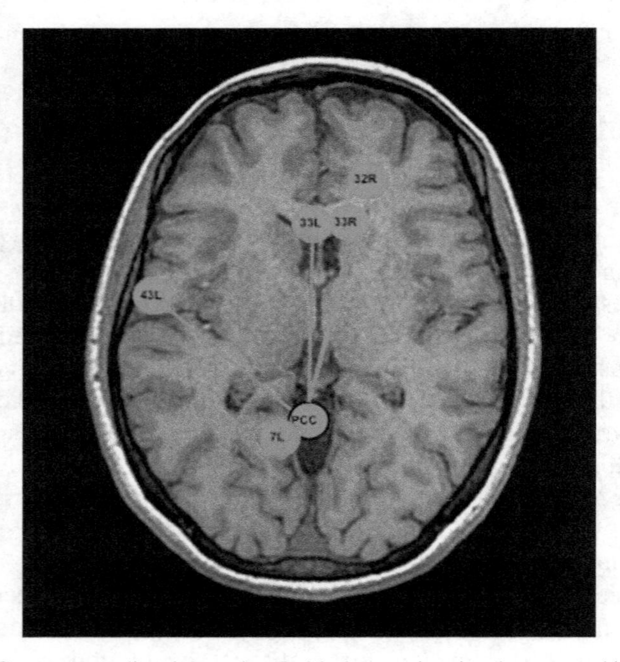

Figure 3.8. The PCC source was directly correlated with the anterior cingulate cortex (right, 33R) ($\beta = 0.16$; $p = 0.02$), anterior cingulate cortex (left, 33L) ($\beta = 0.17$; $p = 0.02$), subcentral area 'gustatory cortical area' (left, 43L) ($\beta = 0.16$; $p = 0.03$), somatosensory associative cortex (left, 7L) ($\beta = 0.13$; $p = 0.03$) and dorsal anterior cingulate cortex (right, 32R) ($\beta = 0.10$; $p = 0.04$).

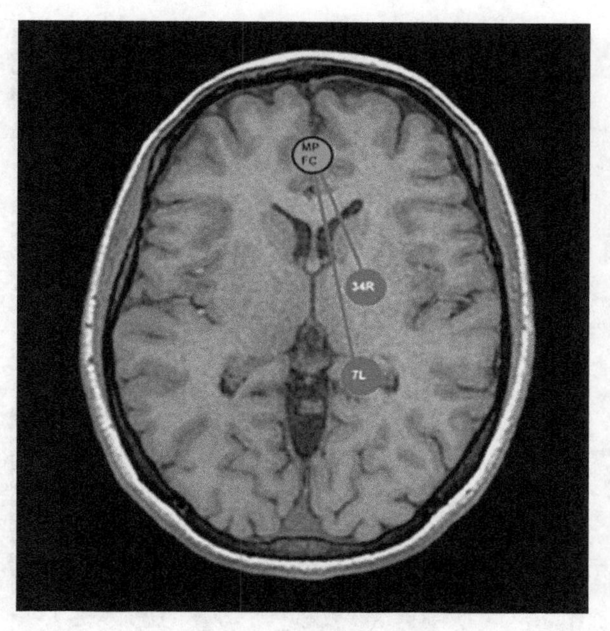

Figure 3.9. The MPFC source was inversely correlated with the somatosensory associative cortex (right, 5R) ($\beta = -0.10$; $p = 0.01$) and anterior entorhinal cortex (right, 34R) ($\beta = -0.10$; $p = 0.03$).

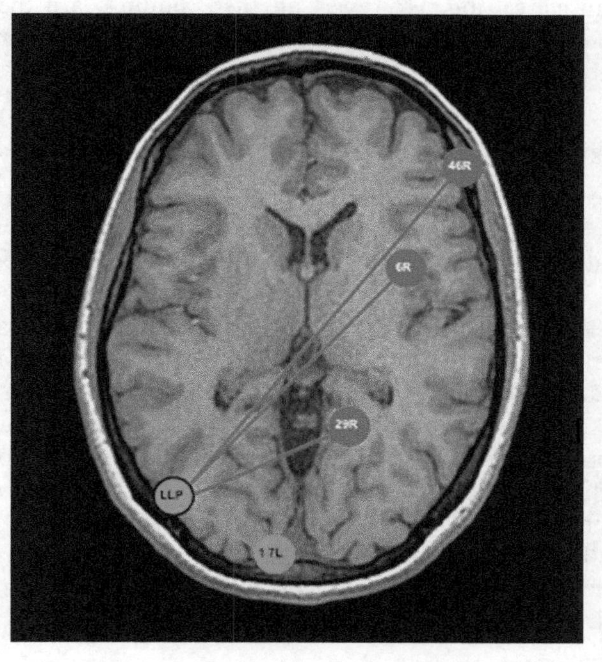

Figure 3.10. The MPFC source was inversely correlated with the somatosensory associative cortex (right, 5R) ($\beta = -0.10$; $p = 0.01$) and anterior entorhinal cortex (right, 34R) ($\beta = -0.10$; $p = 0.03$).

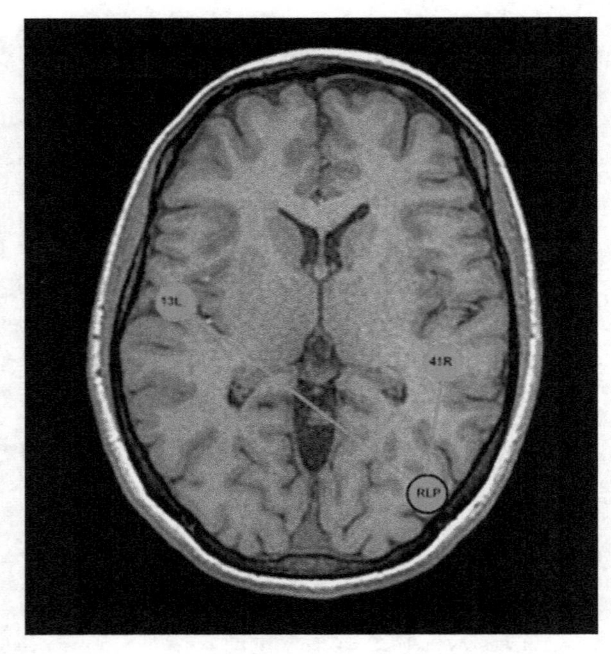

Figure 3.11. RLP source directly correlated with the auditory cortex (right, 41R) ($\beta = 0.19$; $p = 0.04$) and insula cortex (left, 13L) ($\beta = 0.06$; $p = 0.04$).

tastes in a primitive setting. However, all these findings are the basis to understanding differences in the gustatory stimuli in pathological patients and to understanding the pathological origins and implications of these facts.

3.11 Conclusions

Only a small portion of the vast mass of data produced by the fcMRI technique was presented. The correlation between the various areas of the brain when it is carrying out all the vital functions has connected the theory of networks and medicine. Through the theory of networks, the mathematical explanation of some of the most incredible properties of the brain can be introduced. There is still a lot to learn, but the road taken aims to reach a deeper knowledge of brain functioning. The technique of functional magnetic resonance can still improve with the development of technology, and the algorithms for the analysis of the emergent adaptive properties of neuronal networks can still improve, thanks to the continued development of theoretical physics. The application of statistical methods of thermodynamics to describe the behaviour of neurons will give much more information about the nature and the properties of fMRI signal oscillations. fMRI is an efficient tool for diagnosis and it is an innovative field of study for the new generations of medical physicist and physicians.

References

[1] Loscalzo J 2017 *Network Medicine* (Cambridge, MA: Harvard University Press)
[2] Caldarelli G and Catanzaro M 2016 *Scienza delle Reti* (Milan: EGEA SPA)
[3] Barabasi A 2016 *Network Science* (Cambridge: Cambridge University Press)
[4] Saba L 2016 *Magnetic Resonance Imaging Handbook* (Boca Raton, FL: CRC Press)
[5] The MathWorks, MATLAB https://it.mathworks.com/
[6] Friston K J, Ashburner J, Kiebel S J, Nichols T E and Penny W D (ed) 2007 *Statistical Parametric Mapping: The Analysis of Functional Brain Images* (New York: Academic)
[7] Carsetti A 2000 *Functional Models of Cognition* (Berlin: Springer)
[8] Sacks O 1985 *The Man Who Mistook His Wife for a Hat* (New York: Harper and Row)
[9] Biswal B *et al* 1998 Abnormal cerebral activation associated with a motor task in Tourette syndrome *Am. J. Neuroradiol.* **19** 1509–12
[10] Lerner A *et al* 2007 Neuroimaging of neuronal circuits involved in tic generation in patients with Tourette syndrome *Neurology* **68** 1979–87
[11] Church J A *et al* 2009 Control networks in paediatric Tourette syndrome show immature and anomalous patterns of functional connectivity *Brain* **132** 225–38
[12] Fox M D *et al* 2007 Spontaneous fluctuations in brain activity observed with functional magnetic resonance imaging *Nat. Rev. Neurosci.* **8** 700–11
[13] Dosenbach N U F *et al* 2007 Distinct brain networks for adaptive and stable task control in humans *PNAS* **104** 11073–8
[14] Buzsáki G and Draguhn A 2004 Neuronal oscillations in cortical networks *Science* **304** 1926–9
[15] Whitfield-Gabrieli S and Nieto-Castanon A 2012 CONN: a functional connectivity toolbox for correlated and anticorrelated brain networks *Brain Connect.* **2** 125–41
[16] Amaro E Jr and Barker G J 2006 Study design in fMRI: basic principles *Brain Cogn.* **60** 220–2
[17] Forman S D, Cohen J D, Fitzgerald M, Eddy W F, Mintun M A and Noll D C 1995 Improved assessment of significant activation in functional magnetic resonance imaging (fMRI): use of a cluster-size threshold *Magn. Reson. Med.* **33** 636–47
[18] Martuzzi R *et al* 2011 Whole-brain voxel based measure of intrinsic connectivity contrast reveals local changes in tissue connectivity with anesthetic without *a priori* assumptions on thresholds or regions of interest *Neuroimage* **58** 1044–50
[19] Andreoni M, Giacometti A, Maida I, Meraviglia P, Ripamonti D and Sarmati L 2012 HIV–HCV coinfection: epidemiology, pathogenesis and therapeutic implications *Eur. Rev. Med. Pharmacol. Sci.* **16** 1473–83
[20] Biswal B, Yetkin F Z, Haughton V M and Hyde J S 1995 Functional connectivity in the motor cortex of resting human brain using echo-planar MRI *Magn. Reson. Med.* **34** 537–41
[21] Clifford D B and Ances B M 2013 HIV-associated neurocognitive disorder *Lancet Infect. Dis.* **13** 976–86
[22] Masouleh S K *et al* 2017 Functional connectivity alterations in patients with chronic hepatitis C virus infection: a multimodal MRI study *J. Viral Hepat.* **24** 216–25
[23] Plessis S D, Vink M, Joska J A, Koutsilieri E, Stein D J and Emsley R 2014 HIV infection and the frontostriatal system: a systematic review and meta-analysis of fMRI studies *AIDS* **28** 803–11

[24] Qi R *et al* 2013 Altered effective connectivity network of the basal ganglia in low-grade hepatic encephalopathy: a resting-state fMRI study with Granger causality analysis *PLoS One* **8** e53677
[25] Randolph C, Tierney M C, Mohr E and Chase T N 1998 The repeatable battery for the assessment of neuropsychological status (RBANS): preliminary clinical validity *J. Clin. Exp. Neuropsychol.* **20** 310–9
[26] Sollai G 2017 First objective evaluation of taste sensitivity to 6-*n*-propylthiouracil (PROP), a paradigm gustatory stimulus in humans *Sci. Rep.* **7** 40353

IOP Publishing

Neurological Disorders and Imaging Physics, Volume 1
Application of multiple sclerosis
Luca Saba and Jasjit S Suri

Chapter 4

MRI spectroscopy in neurological disorders

Paolo Garofalo, Michele Porcu, Jasjit S Suri, Antonella Balestrieri, Paolo Siotto and Luca Saba

4.1 Introduction

Magnetic resonance spectroscopy (MRS) represents a relatively new, powerful tool in most modern MRI scanners, that provides important clinical information about several diseases. In the early 1950s Proctor noticed that the Larmor frequency of a specific nucleus depends on the molecules in which it is included and he called this effect 'chemical shift' [1]. MRS uses 'chemical shift' to discriminate the biochemical structure and nature of molecules. Although most MRI scanners are set up on the physics of protons (the ^{1}H isotope), which is highly represented in brain tissue, MRS can be applied to virtually any nuclei with non-null magnetic spin, such as fluorine (^{19}F), sodium, carbon (^{13}C) and phosphate (^{31}P) [2]. The choice of one of these nuclei will depend on what biological pathways are to be analyzed. Specific peaks identify each molecule, while the area under the peak corresponds to the number of nuclei analyzed, and hence to their metabolic activity. The most sensitive nucleus is ^{1}H, which shows the highest signal-to-noise ratio in MRS (^{1}H-MRS). In the human brain, ^{1}H-MRS can detect several types of metabolites *in vitro*. *In vivo* ^{1}H-MRS measures only *N*-acetyl-aspartate (NAA), choline (Cho), creatine and phosphocreatine (Cre), lactate (Lac), glutammate, inositol and GABA.

NAA can be considered a neuronal density biomarker due to its high concentration in neurons. Its function in the human brain is not fully understood, but many studies conducted in rats have revealed that it is a polypeptide synthetized from aspartate and acetyl-coenzyme A into mitochondria [3]. Despite NAA being mainly an intra-neural biomarker, it can also be found in oligodendroglia precursors and it plays many roles, such as: a cotransport substrate for molecular water pumps, avoiding osmotic shock in neurons, an energetic reservoir of glutammate and a precursor of NAAG, derived from glutammate and NAA. NAAG is the most diffuse cerebral dipeptide serving as a neurostimulator in neurons, oligodendrocytes and microglia [4]. The Cho signal reflects levels of mobile choline, including choline,

doi:10.1088/2053-2563/ab1fdcch4

acetylcholine and phospho-choline (a precursor of phosphatidylcholine), and high levels of choline are related to an increase of cellular replication or cell membrane destruction. Inositol is a biomarker of glial cell density. Lac is the product of anaerobic glycolysis under hypoxic–ischemic conditions. The peak of Cr reflects cellular metabolic reserves, due to creatinine and phosphocreatine [5].

The first clinical *in vivo* application of ^{1}H-MRS was on the human brain [6]. In particular, MRS can support the imaging assessment of many neurological disorders. MRS can be useful in the assessment of hypoxic–ischemic injuries, neoplastic disease, epilepsy, and inflammatory, infective, metabolic and degenerative disorders.

The purpose of this chapter is to give a brief description of the main useful target-points to consider in MR spectra for the evaluation and characterization of neurological diseases.

4.2 Magnetic resonance spectroscopy and hypoxic–ischemic conditions

Hypoxic–ischemic encephalopathy (HIE) results from a deficient supply of oxygen to the brain tissues. This condition results in functional cognitive impairment that leads to severe neurodevelopmental disabilities and long-term deficits in children [7, 8]. Conventional MRI, conducted with T1-weighted images, inversion recovery-weighted images, T2-weighted images or diffusion weighted images (DWIs) including an apparent diffusion coefficient (ADC) map, shows two typical distribution patterns of lesions:

(1) The *watershed pattern* involves specific white matter territories located into the vascular 'watershed zone' of the brain [9].
(2) The *nucleo-capsular pattern* involves deep gray matter and the peri-rolandic cortex and may extend to the entire cortex [9].

The most common appearance on conventional MRI sequences of hypoxic–ischemic injury persisting for more than ten minutes is restricted diffusion on DWI and ADC maps, subtle hyperintensity on T1-weighted image that may extend two days after birth or later, while T2-weighted image results are negative [10].

^{1}H-MRS is a proven MRI tool in the assessment of HIE [11]. While conventional MRI and DWI imaging can show false negative results, ^{1}H-MRS shows more sensitivity in detecting injury in the first 24 h after a hypoxic–ischemic event [12]. Since ischemic changes are more evident and severe in the cortex than in white matter, spectral evaluation is primarily conducted by a single-voxel, located in the occipital cortex, basal ganglia and watershed zones [13]. The main spectral findings in the basal ganglia and watershed zones during ischemic injuries concern the reduction of the peaks of NAA and NAA/Cr, in particular in subacute and chronic settings [14]. Some authors consider the reduction of the NAA level and NAA/Cr as the most the important elements to determine prognosis [15]. Within three days of the ischemic insult and hypoxic injuries, myo-inositol and choline peaks are normal, while an increase of Cho/Cr with subsequent reduction of Cr relates to a high grade of injury and poor outcome [15]. Other important spectra to analyze are Lac, glutamine/glutamate (Glx) and lipids.

Lac is the main biomarker associated with hypoxia and its level is typically higher in the early stages, within two to eight hours after insult [13]. An abnormal increase of the lactate peak is the most common consequence of anaerobic glycolysis and it occurs twice during ischemic injury. The first peak occurs after the event and incipient hypoxemia. The second peak, over the following 24–48 h, is a result of secondary energy failure; in this condition, the 'surviving' neurons start to deplete their energetic storage because of mitochondrial failure. The detection and quantification of the lactate range requires a long TE because of the long T2 relaxation time of lactate. The adoption of short TE sequences can lead to an overlap with lipid spectra and alter its estimate [13]. A major pitfall to consider is that preterm infants can show slightly higher physiological levels of lactate in the watershed regions without evidence of ischemic conditions [12].

Glutamine/Glutamate levels reflect brain activity, so they can be sensitive but unreliable markers to estimate the gravity of oxygen depletion.

Lipid levels are considered to be associated with other altered metabolite spectra reflecting poor outcomes. As an isolated parameter, lipid changes relate to better outcomes.

The NAA level and NAA/Cr are typically normal, compared to lactate, in the first three days after ischemic injury, while they are preferred indicators of the gravity of insult in the late stages. Despite these findings, some authors consider increased lactate/choline of up to 1 as being related to the poorest outcomes for ischemic injuries [16].

4.3 Magnetic resonance spectroscopy and neoplastic disease

While conventional MRI is a corroborated method to investigate the morphology of brain tumors, MRS is becoming the most useful tool to determine the metabolic profile of tumors in clinical practice. Many *in vivo* studies of MRS have been used to characterize tumors and tumor-like lesions [17], but the primary roles of this method in a diagnostic setting of this class of neurologic pathology are:

- Monitoring low-grade tumors after surgery and radiotherapy.
- Distinguishing non-necrotic from necrotic neoplastic areas to guide stereotaxic biopsy procedures.
- Guiding neurosurgeons through the radical excision of tumors located in eloquent brain areas.

Neoplastic tissues present altered biological pathways and MRS allows one to study the metabolomics of tumors through the analysis of the principal metabolites involved in these pathways [18]. The first characteristic of a neoplastic cell's phenotype is the alteration of oxidative metabolism that leads to enhanced lactic acid production causing intracellular acidosis [19]. To balance the intracellular storage of protons, cells upregulate the activity of the transmembrane Na^+/K^+ charger and carbonic anhydrase, leading to massive extrusion of H^+ in the extracellular space with a relative increase of intracellular pH [20]. The alkaline intracellular pH supports proliferation, while extracellular acidosis sustains neo-angiogenetic processes [20]. Neoplastic cells have very high energy consumption to sustain vital activities and provide proteins and nucleotides for their replication. Suppression of oxidative metabolism in favor of lactate causes a decrease of mitochondrial function and then to lower levels of high energy phosphates such as ATP and phosphocreatine [21]. The overexpressed glycolytic process provides synthesis of proteins and nucleotides derived from intermediate products, such as the amino acid serine that is converted into glycine by the enzyme serine hydroxi-methyltransferase [22]. *In vivo* ^{1}H-MRS can quantify glycine, considered as a biomarker of enhanced glycolysis and nucleotide synthesis of neoplastic cells such as malignant glioma [23]. Myo-inositol (MI) is a metabolite involved in the maintenance of the integrity of the cellular membrane in reactive astrocytes and an increase of MI typically relates to astrocytic proliferation and demyelination processes [24]. Therefore, the MI spectrum will be higher in tumors and multiple sclerosis, but lower in Alzheimer's disease (AD), sclerosis tuberosa (ST), and other metabolic and inflammatory white matter diseases [25]. The choline signal increases in tumor tissues due to rapid cellular proliferation [26]. In contrast to a decrease of NAA, due to neuronal loss, Cho/NAA becomes much more important as biomarker of tumor tissue detected in MRS. The 'Kennedy pathway' governs the turnover of phospholipids [27]. This pathway describes the synthesis of phosphatidylcholine via choline and phosphor-choline and its breakdown into glycerol–phosphor-choline. ^{1}H-MRS can measure phospholipids through total choline levels intended as the sum of all these elements and cannot differentiate among them. In particular, P-Cho is a metabolite derived from phosphorylation of choline by choline-kinase-α, an intracellular enzyme upregulated in malignant variants of glioma [28]. Increased P-Cho/GPC represents a biomarker of a malignant variant of glial brain tumor compared to a low-grade tumor [29]. Primary neuro-glial cell tumors represent the main field of clinical application for MRS [30]. In particular, glioblastoma multi-forme (GBM) is the most malignant form of cerebral neoplasm (figure 4.1) originating from astrocytes that could be well investigated with routine morpho-logical MRI [31]. Structural imaging reveals a poorly demarcated mass with cystic elements, necrotic degeneration and infiltrating edema [31]. Cross-sectional patho-logical examination shows different crammed cell types, focal necrosis and dense microvascular networks, both inside and near the neoplastic mass relate to high-grade malignancy [30]. A major problem in prognostic work-up is the delineation of the tumor border zone. MRI cannot clearly visualize these regions and they represent the main cause of tumor recurrence after surgical and radiotherapy treatments [32]. To face this issue, recent research, published by Martinez-Bisbal and colleagues, tried to combine classical morphological MRI with a ^{1}H-MRS study of a neoplastic sample to obtain a structural combination of chemical, cyto-architectural and vascular features [33]. In this experimental *ex vivo* study, morphological evaluation of the samples of GBM was conducted using multislice three-plane RARE sequences, while PRESS sequences with single and multivoxel acquisitions for spectroscopy evaluation on a 14 T magnet were used. The results

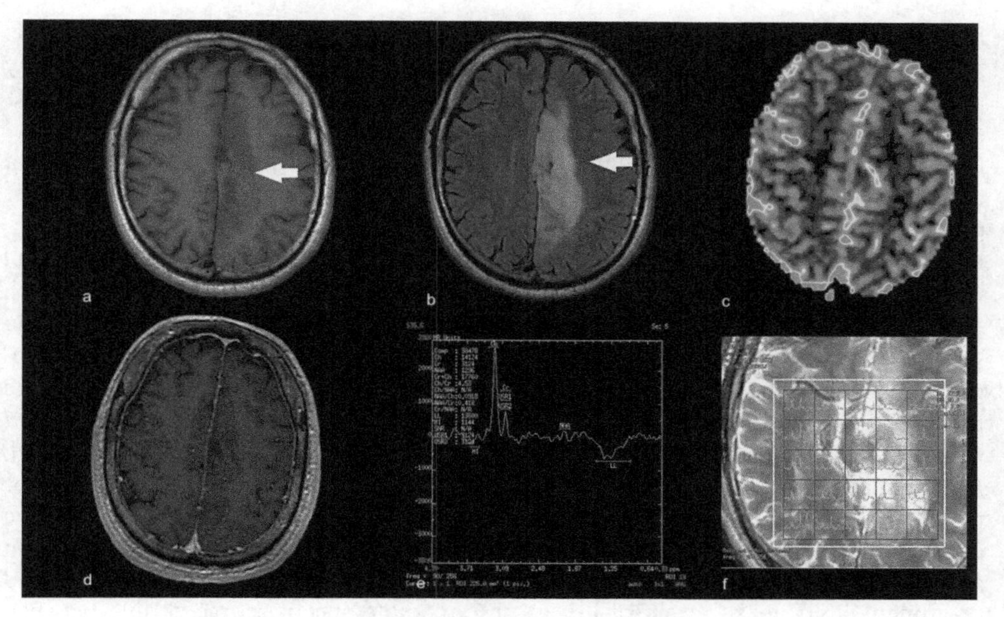

Figure 4.1. Brain neoplasm in a 57-year-old male patient.

showed high-grade overlapping between pathological examinations and structural images. The spectroscopy analysis of the metabolites of the samples was characteristic, detecting neoplasm in spared brain tissue. In particular, ^{1}H-MRS provided a metabolic profile including Lac, Cr, Cho, Glx, NAA and Alanine. This analysis showed a different distribution of some of these metabolites:

- NAA was higher outside the tumor tissue.
- Cho was higher near the periphery of the tumor.
- Cr was low inside the neoplastic mass.
- Lac was exclusively present inside the tumor.

Furthermore, ^{1}H-MRS is a useful tool to study pH in neoplastic tissue. It reveals the low value of pH in the non-viable portion of the tumor, while high values of pH are present in the viable part of the tumor [34]. The metabolomics of glucose is also peculiar in the neoplasm, since glucose shows a higher concentration in the tumor due to the maximal capacity of the cellular glucose cotransport carrier [35, 36].

MRS alone cannot depict a specific brain tumor because many spectroscopic patterns are heterogeneous and common to many histological types of tumors. Therefore, this is the method of choice to show the heterogeneous distribution of metabolites across a neoplasm. Glial family tumors are the only class to show a characteristic *in vivo* spectroscopic pattern. In particular, they present low levels of NAA and high levels of total Cho (t-Cho), respectively, reflecting the loss of neuronal tissue and higher membrane turnover with cellular density. Nevertheless, despite their utility in a diagnostic setting, these values are misleading. In fact, many neuronal diseases, such as encephalitis or cerebritis, tumefactive demyelination lesions or infarction, can alter NAA levels. In contrast, regular levels of t-Cho inside the neoplasm will exclude any malignant switch, whereas high levels are usually present in pilocytic astrocytoma, encephalitis, active dismyelination process, TBC and post-irradiation injuries [37]. Another misleading signal is from lipids, derived from microscopic and intracellular lipids presence in high-grade tumors without a clear necrotic process. Myo-inositol and creatine are highly represented both in low-grade astrocytoma, gliomatosis cerebri and demyelination processes. In particular, high intra-lesion levels of myo-inositol support low-grade glioma diagnosis [38] while a higher creatine concentration relates to shorter progression-free survival [39].

The most important role of proton spectroscopy is indeed to differentiate low-grade from high-grade glioma and discriminate astrocytoma from oligodendroglioma. To simplify this process, many studies, rather than considering single metabolites, have adopted ratios between them, such as Cho/NAA and NAA/Cho, increasing the reproducibility and sensitivity of the measures [40]. Furthermore, ^{1}H-MRS shows a characteristic pattern of chemical profiles for primary CNS lymphoma (PCNSL), brain metastasis (BM) and other specific entities, such as primitive neuro-ectodermal tumors (PNET), meningioma and brain abscess. Enhancing the central area of PCNSL shows a mild increase of t-Cho and prominent lipid peaks at short TE, an intermediate spectroscopic profile between high-grade glioma and BM [41]. According to their different histologies, the BM profile could be very heterogeneous, as a proliferating solid BM typically shows an elevated peak of Cho with higher Cho/NAA than the infiltrating glioma, whereas a necrotic BM presents high lactate and lipid peaks [42]. Medulloblastoma is a very rare neoplastic entity of the PNET family, mostly recurrent in childhood, which presents high levels of some specific metabolites, such as taurine, an organic amino acid involved in many biological functions [43]. Less specific is the spectroscopic profile of meningioma. This class of neoplasms has many different histologic patterns and the utility of ^{1}H-MRS is limited to identifying alanine, a non-specific biomarker that is also present in abscesses together with other amino acids, which increase due to enhanced glycolysis and then high levels of pyruvate. Since recurrent tumors often occur in the marginal zone, ^{1}H-MRS plays another important role in the therapeutic setting of brain neoplasms, i.e. the sampling of peripheral enhancing border-zone regions. Many studies have confirmed increased t-Cho levels and elevated Cho/NAA in these regions and surrounding tissues. Thus, ^{1}H-MRS sampling would help achieve much prolonged progression-free survival for high-grade gliomas [44].

Another relevant function of MRS in the daily management of brain tumors is treatment monitoring after radiation and chemotherapy regimes. Although both radiotherapy- and chemotherapy-induced brain injuries do not have any spectroscopic matching data on proton spectroscopy due to low spectral quality [45], phosphorus spectroscopy might be more specific and less prone to spectral artifacts in detecting the difference between phosphor-monoesters and phosphor-diesters.

4.4 Magnetic resonance spectroscopy and epilepsy

The main purpose of MRI imaging in epilepsy is to find the underlying cause of epileptic focus and detect any treatable epileptogenic lesions such as vascular malformations, cerebral hematoma, brain tumors, congenital malformations or inborn errors of metabolism.

MRS enhances the information on metabolic derangements, such as creatine deficiency, and mitochondrial disorders occurring in epilepsy. Furthermore, together with structural MRI, MRS helps in the differential diagnosis and characterization between focal cortical dysplasia (FCD) and neoplasia. Seizures typically cause an increase of the metabolic demands on brain tissue, because of the elevated and chaotic electrical activity of neurons, leading to abnormal levels of Lac and a reduction of NAA [46]. The most common causes of childhood onset epilepsy are mitochondrial and metabolic disorders [47]. In particular, mitochondrial disorders show heterogeneous phenotypes with partial or generalized forms of epilepsy [48]. Bianchi *et al* noticed that normal-appearing white or gray matter in structural MRI might hide an abnormal spectroscopic profile of metabolites [49]. The researchers performed, in an epileptic cohort of pediatric patients, single-voxel MRS sampling on normal-appearing peritrigonal and cerebellar white matter and cortical gray matter, and observed reduction of Cho and Cr peaks together with abnormal NAA/Cr and Lac levels [49]. Cr reflects an important neuronal energetic reserve, and L-arginine-glycine amidinotransferase (AGAT) and guanidinoacetatemethyltransferase (GAMT) with the SLC6A8 transporter control its intra–extra neuronal balance. Cr reduction is usually due to a genetic deficiency of the enzymes and cellular carrier and its deficiency is present in many other diseases such as mental retardation and autism [50]. Another important cause of inborn drug-resistant epilepsy is FCD type II [51]. FCD includes a wide spectrum of malformations, characterized by Taylor in the early 1870s by the presence of ectopic nervous tissue in otherwise normal white matter. The International League Against Epilepsy (ILAE) classified three different pathologic types of FCD, distinguishing isolated forms (type I and II) from those associated with other principal lesions. In particular, FCD type I is a derangement into an abnormal radial (Ia), tangential (Ib) or mixed (Ic) cortical lamination, FCD type II contains dysmorphic neurons (IIa) or dysmorphic neurons and balloon cells (IIb), and FCD type III contains deranged cortical lamination associated with temporal-hippocampal sclerosis (IIIa) or glial oligo-glial tumor (IIIb) with no vascular malformation (IIIc) or any other acquired lesions. Many studies have confirmed a reproducible spectroscopic pattern in the brain with FCD showing an alteration of NAA, Cho and Cr levels [52]. Some authors, using high-field 3 T MRS, found a significant increase of Cho and reduction of NAA spectra among patients with FCD type II [53]. These alterations are explicable by an altered architecture of brain tissue containing immature and undifferentiated neurons, in addition to cell loss and associated gliosis, and help to distinguish FCD from brain neoplasia, which shows reduced NAA/Cr [54]. Despite decreased NAA/Cr being common in both FCD and brain neoplasia, the relatively normal level of Cho/Cr in FCD may help in differential diagnosis when conventional MRI is not sufficient. In this perspective, MRS represents a reliable tool, together with clinical examination and EEG semiology, in pre-operative mapping of epileptogenic 'nidus'. In this specific setting, Cendes [55] and Kuzniecky [56] used NAA/Cr as a biomarker of epileptogenic nidus in refractory TLE, with 87% greater sensibility than morphologic MRI.

Another useful application in the clinical management of epilepsy is the monitoring of the response to antiepileptic drug (AED) therapy. In particular, as demonstrated by Campos *et al*, MRS can predict the response among patients with temporal lobe epilepsy, showing a significant reduction of NAA/Cr in the hippocampi [57].

4.5 Magnetic resonance spectroscopy and inflammatory disease of the central nervous system

Inflammatory pathology of the central nervous system (CNS) embraces many different diseases. They relate to a wide range of humoral and cellular responses to external factors, such as infection or post-traumatic events. Moreover, autoimmunity and degenerative disorders come from the same cause. The blood–brain barrier (BBB) rules out the existing interactions between the immune system and brain and its breakdown represents the pathologic substrate of neuro-inflammation leading to neuronal damage and then to repair processes including neurogenesis [58]. These phenomena result in the acute release of cytokines and chemokines, causing local vasodilatation with exudate, tissue damage and neuronal apoptosis followed by chronic milder inflammatory reaction with secondary activation of astrocytes and repair processes [59]. Therefore, the primary role of MRI in inflammatory disease of the CNS is to study the BBB with related white matter damage and MRS could give additional value in the evaluation of the etiology of these changes, helping in the differential diagnostic process.

4.5.1 MRS and demyelination disorders

Multiple sclerosis (MS) represents the most common demyelinating disorder of the CNS. The clinical patterns of MS progression are very different: relapsing–remitting, primary progressive, progressive relapsing and secondary progressive [60]. The pathologic basis of MS depends on demyelination with secondary aberrant re-myelination and gliosis with or without axonal destruction [61]. MRI is a suitable tool to observe the spatial and temporal dissemination of MS lesions and it is a highly standardized method to evaluate and stage the severity and progression of disease in accordance with recent updates of McDonald's criteria [62]. MRS has become an integral part of the imaging management of MS, and is applied to detect early lesions and differentiate them from other similar lesions [63]. In particular, acute lesions show decreased signals of the NAA spectrum because of axonal injuries and secondary loss with a later partial recovery of its levels, in parallel to clinical improvement [64]. Other important biomarkers in acute phase MS are increased levels of Cho, associated with glial proliferation or myelin breakdown [65], elevated levels of Glx, indicating excitotoxic effects secondary to axonal injury and increased

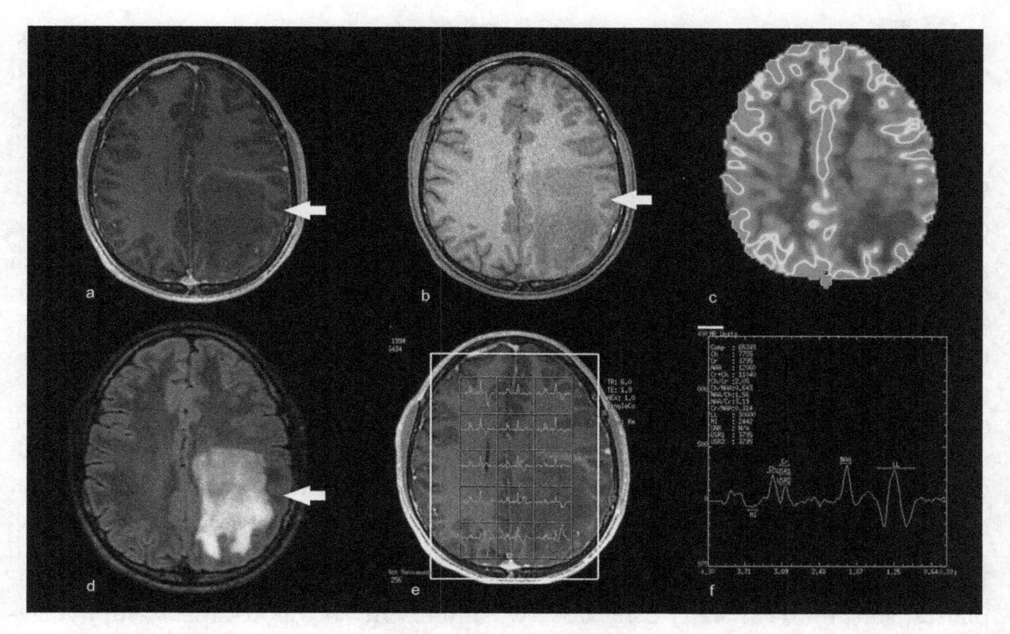

Figure 4.2. Pseudotumoral lesion in a 38-year-old male patient with multiple sclerosis.

levels of lactate related to non-specific inflammatory process. The reduction of macromolecule peaks at 0.9 and 1.3 ppm represents the most reliable marker of acute damage of myelin with secondary release of myelin fragments [66]. During the chronic phase of MS, MRS shows progressive normalization of levels of Cho and Lac while myo-inositol levels, related to glial proliferation, remain elevated (figure 4.2) [64]. Together with these results, many studies on cortical gray matter have demonstrated different patterns of these metabolites in ^{1}H-MRS. In particular, Kapeller *et al* [67] observed decreased levels of myo-inositol in cortical gray matter while other researchers noticed a reduction of NAA, Cho and Glx among MS patients within normal-appearing gray matter, compared to healthy subjects. Additionally, ^{1}H-MRS may contribute to the assessment of clinical functional recovery and related degree of disability, through an estimate of changes in NAA/Cr as indirect expression of cortical damage [63]. Furthermore, relapsing–remitting MS patients present significantly changed levels of myo-inositol and Glx in normal-appearing white matter as expression of clinical overcome [68].

Acute disseminated encephalomyelitis (ADEM) is an acute monophasic inflammatory demyelinating disease affecting CNS [69]. The recognition of the early signs of ADEM and its differential diagnosis from other demyelinating diseases represents a crucial step to assess the correct therapeutic management of patients with early anti-inflammatory treatment. In this vein, ^{1}H-MRS may help the diagnostic process of differentiating demyelinating tumefactive brain lesions from neoplasm showing different patterns of metabolites. In particular, Cianfoni and colleagues observed high peaks of glutamate and glutamine as specific markers of demyelinating diseases as compared to aggressive intra-axial neoplasm, in which they observed non-specific signs such as: reduction of NAA levels, indicating neuronal loss; elevated Cho levels, reflecting elevated cellular turnover; and reduced levels of Cr, reflecting depressed cellular energetics or cellular death [70].

4.5.2 MRS and infective disorders

CNS infections represent an important cause of neurological disability and, if not promptly treated, they can be life-threatening. MRI and advanced techniques, such as MRS, allow accurate diagnosis and improve the characterization of focal or diffuse infectious lesions, differentiating them from other types of CNS lesions [71]. CNS infections are usually of bacterial origin. Bacterial abscesses are frequently secondary to direct extensions from head and neck infectious processes, such as sinusitis, mastoiditis, meningitis or dental abscesses, or they derive from hematic spread from an extra-cranial location, for example a lung or urinary tract infection or endocarditis. The most common bacterial agents involved in immunocompetent adults are *Streptococcus spp* and *Staphylococcus aureus. Klebsiella* is common in diabetic patients while fungi such as *Aspergillus* and *Nocardia* are common in transplant patients [72]. The pathologic evolution of brain abscesses occurs in four phases, starting from 'early cerebritis', which presents as a non-capsulated, hyperemic and edematous mass with hypo- to isointensity in T1W, homogeneous hyperintensity in T2W and diffusion restriction in DWIs. The subsequent 'late cerebritis' phase shows stronger but irregular rim enhancement after contrast medium administration and presents a hyperintense core in T2W and FLAIR sequences, and iso- to mildly hyperintense in T1W. The abscess capsule appears as a thin, complete but irregular hypointense rim in T2W and hypointense in T1W and it takes up a lot of contrast medium. Later, the rim-enhancing capsule becomes thicker [73]. MRS plays an important role in narrowing differential diagnosis among other ring-enhancing lesions. In particular, MRS shows the elevation of the succinate peak (at 2.40 ppm) and high lactate (at 1.33 ppm), acetate (at 1.92 ppm), alanine (at 1.47 ppm), valine, leucine and isoleucine levels (at 0.9 ppm) may be present. Cho, Cr and NAA peaks are reduced or not detected at all [74]. The potential role of MRS is to differentiate between aerobic and anaerobic abscesses, showing lower acetate and succinate peaks in aerobic than anaerobic abscesses [75]. Additional important information is the presence of amino acids in the spectra, which narrows the differential diagnosis between an abscess and necrotic brain tumors [76]. *Mycobacterium tuberculosis* complex represents a very rare but potentially life-threatening source of infection of the CNS. It is relatively common among children and adults who are HIV positive (1% of prevalence) [77]. Tubercoloma is a well-defined focal mass, which appears with a caseation or not-caseation core secondary to hematogenous or cerebrospinal spreading of *M. tuberculosis.* The caseation tubercoloma appears as hypo- to isointense in T1W and iso- to hypointense in T2W sequences with ring enhancement. A non-caseation tubercoloma instead appears as hypointense in T1W and hyperintense in T2W sequences [78]. MRS may show characteristic high levels of lipid peaks distinguishing tubercoloma from abscesses and brain tumors [79].

Herpes virus complex represents the most common cause of acquired viral infections of the CNS. Herpes simplex virus (HSV) infection can be congenital or acquired. HSV shows particular tropism for the limbic system (i.e. temporal lobes, insular cortex, sub-frontal area and cingulate gyri); extra-limbic involvement is more common in childhood. Pathologic features, such as petechial hemorrhages with massive necrosis and cerebral edema, are very common and they are accompanied by neuronophagia, apoptosis and tissue destruction [80]. MRI is the method of choice to correctly assess viral infection of the CNS. T1W sequences show cortical swelling and reducing contrast intensity at gray–white interfaces. T2W scans show isolated gray matter hyperintensity with relative sparing of white matter. T2* and susceptibility weighted sequences (SWI or GRE) may show better hemorrhagic foci as focal punctate hypointense areas. DWIs demonstrate cortical restricted diffusion from the early phase of viral infection with coexistent intense gyriform enhancement after contrast medium administration. MRS findings are very typical with reduced NAA, NAA/Cho and NAA/Cr, and are rarely associated with late normalization of NAA/Cr after one year [81]. In HIV encephalitis, early MRI findings are cortical atrophy with focal punctate or patchy white matter damage visible as a hyperintense area on T2 and FLAIR sequences [82]. MRS may show earlier reversible metabolic anomalies in normal-appearing gray and white matter, including elevated signals of Cho and mI and a reduced NAA signal on the frontal cortex and later on the centrum semiovale [83]. MRS can provide useful information about eventual opportunistic infections occurring in HIV patients, assisting differential diagnosis. In particular, neuro toxoplasmosis typically shows elevated levels of lipids and cryptococcosis is associated with high levels of both lactate and lipids to 0.9 ppm with decreased resonance peaks of Cho, Cr and NAA [84]. Brain lymphoma is a possible but fortunately not frequent eventuality for HIV patients. Spectral analysis of this post-infective neoplasia shows elevated Cho and lipid signals, although lower than for toxoplasmosis [85].

4.6 Magnetic resonance spectroscopy and metabolic disorders

Metabolic disorders are relatively uncommon neurological illnesses. We can classify them as acquired and inherited, but they are now understood to be linked, because many exogenous agents show a direct mutagen effect on the brain, leading to toxic storage of metabolites. Both inherited and acquired metabolic disorders predominantly affect deep gray matter nuclei, in accordance with their high metabolic activity, and white matter with a bilateral symmetric pattern. Conventional MRI provides the locations of these lesions, although many MRI signal abnormalities may overlap, showing the same lesion patterns for different diseases. Advanced MRI techniques, such as MRS, may assist in differential diagnosis, giving a quantitative evaluation of the extent of neuronal damage with relative impairment and brain degeneration.

The most common acquired metabolic disorders of the CNS are hepatic encephalopathy, hypoglycemic encephalopathy and alcohol related encephalopathy (Wernicke encephalopathy).

Hepatic encephalopathy represents a common secondary acquired metabolic disorder of the CNS secondary to acute or chronic failure of the liver [86]. A lack of hepatic metabolism leads to toxic blood levels of ammonia and other metabolites, such as manganese, with osmotic swelling of astrocytes following glutamine intracellular accumulation and an increase of inhibitory neurotransmitter synthesis [87]. Conventional MRI shows the typical involvement of both cortico-spinal tracts, with bilateral hyperintensity in T2-FLAIR sequences. Other T2-FLAIR hyperintense foci may be seen in the thalamic and cortical cortex, periventricular white matter and in the posterior limb of the internal capsule [86]. Manganese shows a more peculiar behavior than ammonia, showing tropism for the globus pallidus, substantia nigra, tectal plate, hypothalamus and pituitary gland. In these regions, the pathologic storage of this metal appears as T1W hyperintense areas in accordance with its different paramagnetic behavior [88]. MRS may narrow the differential diagnosis of hepatic encephalopathy, revealing a specific pattern of glutamine and glutamate increased peaks, with a compensative decrease of Cho and mI [88]. After liver transplantation, MRS shows the restoration of the normal appearance of spectra in affected brain areas [89].

Hypoglycemic encephalopathy is another common cause of acquired metabolic disease of the CNS, secondary to anti-diabetic drug therapy or hidden releasing insulinoma, following rapid decrease of hematic levels of glucose below 50 mg dL^{-1} [90, 91]. The sudden reduction of glucose leads to abnormal function, even to failure, of neuronal ATPase with consequent release of aspartate and other excitatory neurotransmitters that cause toxic effects to the cerebral cortex, neostriatum and limbic system, with relative sparing of the brainstem and cerebellum [92]. Milder hypoglycemia may affect different brain areas such as the splenium of the corpus callosum, internal capsule and corona radiata [92]. The conventional MRI appearance of hypoglycemic encephalopathy is bilateral and symmetric T2W white matter hyperintensity with reversible restricted diffusion on deep or cortical gray matter of the aforementioned brain areas [93]. Identifying clinical suspects and their correct metabolic assessment is the first step to accurate diagnosis of hypoglycemic encephalopathy and MRS can play a role showing reduced peaks of lactate [93].

Wernicke's encephalopathy (WE) is secondary to thiamine (vitamin B1) deficit [94]. The typical clinical onset of WE is an alteration of consciousness associated with altered gait and sensorium and ocular paresis [94]. Thiamine deficiency is commonly observed in both alcoholics and non-alcoholics as a consequence of malabsorption and bowel malignancy, or it can arise from systemic infection, hyperemesis or prolonged starvation with secondary altered water balance and nutritional deficit [94]. Lack of vitamin B1 leads to neuronal intra and extracellular osmotic swelling, in particular along the periventricular regions [95]. Conventional MRI depicts two patterns of lesion distributions, appearing as hyperintense areas on T2W sequences—typical and atypical. A typical pattern of distribution, common to alcoholics, involves the medial thalami, mamillary bodies, periaqueductal region, tectal plate and floor of the fourth ventricle, while an atypical pattern of distribution, common to non-alcoholics, involves the cerebellum, brainstem nuclei of the VI, VII, VIII and XII cranial nerves, caudate, splenium of the corpus callosum and cerebral cortex [96]. After gadolinium-chelate intravenous administration, these areas may assume light contrast enhancement and this can be the only clear feature of the disease [96]. In this setting, MRS can show similar patterns in the alcoholic and non-alcoholic forms of WE showing reduced levels of NAA and Cr and increased levels of Lac within thalamus and cerebellum with partial recovery after treatment with thiamine [97, 98].

Inherited metabolic encephalopathies (IME) refer to a heterogeneous group of diseases in which genetic derangement, with a subsequent lack of a enzyme or non-enzyme protein, leads to defects in the pathways of synthesis, storage, transport and degradation of metabolic products of neurons and/or glial cells. IMEs comprise four subclasses:

- Disorders due to accumulation of toxic compounds, such as maple syrup urine syndrome and phenylketonuria.
- Disorders due to deficient energy production, such as mitochondrial defects and creatine deficiency.
- Disorders due to altered lysosomial and peroxisomal catabolism of molecules, such as Gaucher or Zellweger disease.
- Disorders involving the metabolism of neurotransmitters, such as glycine and serine.

Conventional MRI rarely helps the neuro-radiologist to narrow these different diagnostic hypotheses clearly, therefore MRS could represent an effective diagnostic tool for these disorders, showing most common spectral alterations.

Maple syrup urine syndrome is an autosomal recessive disorder caused by mitochondrial genetic mutation of an alpha-ketoacid dehydrogenase complex with an altered urea cycle and secondary storage of branched chain amino acids [99]. MRI shows a non-specific hyperintensity pattern with sharp margins on T2-FLAIR sequences, reflecting cerebral edema, within the basal ganglia, posterior limb of internal capsule, brainstem, cerebral peduncles, cerebellum and cerebral hemisphere in newborns. MRS shows a peak at 0.9 ppm due to the storage of branched chains of alpha-ketoacid, visible at short, intermediate and long PRESS MRS acquisition. Some authors have also reported a peak of lactate [100].

Phenylketonuria is a common hereditary metabolic disorder, and is due to mutation in the phenylalanine hydroxylase codifying gene with a subsequent increase of circulating phenylalanine. Phenylalanine (Phe) is a life-long toxic agent to myelogenesis and high levels can cause developmental brain errors in neonates. MRI may reveal nothing. Some cases can be associated with non-specific periventricular, peritrigonal and frontal patchy and irregular white matter hyperintensity on T2-FLAIR sequences, and DWI can show restricted diffusion in these areas as a sign of the progression of disease [101]. MRS reflects a peak of Phe at 7.37 ppm parallel to its normal appearance at 4 ppm on routine MRS [101]. Therefore, this technique is useful to monitor dietary effects and Phe kinetics.

Creatine deficiency syndromes arise from synthesis and transport defects of Cre caused by genetic congenital errors to the GAMT, AGAT and cellular transporter (SLC6A8) transcribing codons [102]. In these patients, MRI usually shows variable

T2-FLAIR hyperintensity and restricted diffusion within the globi pallidi. MRS allows diagnosis when MRI is normal, in particular in children with unexplained hypotonia, showing a reduction of spectra of Cre at 2 ppm in these areas [102].

The *Zellweger syndrome spectrum* include a small range of rare hereditary metabolic diseases including Zellweger syndrome, neonatal adrenoleukodystrophy and infantile Refsum disease. These syndromes are autosomal recessive disorders caused by mutation in the PFXs peroxisome genes and the most common MRI features are abnormal myelination, and micro- and pachygyria with bilateral parasylvian lesions. Hypomyelination is often identified as a large and confluent hyperintense area on T2-FLAIR sequences with an associated sub-ependymal caudo-thalamic germinolytic cyst. MRS shows a lipid peak between 0.8 and 1.33 ppm, a reduced peak of NAA and an increased peak of Cho [103].

Mitochondrial disorders include many rare genetic diseases (Leigh syndrome, MELAS, Kearns–Sayre syndrome and MERRF syndrome) affecting organs with high metabolic activity such as the brain, muscles and bones. MRI and MRS are crucial to ascertain the correct genesis of this class of diseases of the brain. In particular, conventional MRI may overlap, showing the same pattern of bilateral basal ganglia capsular hyperintensity and MRS becomes useful when MRI results are normal, as MRS can show abnormal high levels of Lac and reduction of NAA in deep gray and white matter [104].

4.7 Magnetic resonance spectroscopy and neurodegenerative disorders

The spectrum of neurodegenerative disorders comprises a very wide range of pathologies which have many etiologies. The most common causes of cognitive impairment are primitive, such as Alzheimer's disease (AD) and dementia with Lewy body (DLB), whereas frontotemporal dementia (FTD) and corticobasal degeneration (CBD) are less common. The causes of acquired dementia include acute and chronic cerebrovascular disease with multiple microinfarcts, microbleeds and white matter lesions, and intracranial mass lesions, infections and inflammatory conditions [105]. Less frequent genetic causes of CNS neurodegeneration with secondary dementia are Huntington's disease (HD) and amyotrophic lateral sclerosis (ALS).

Pathologic biomarkers of neurodegeneration in normal age-related brain dementia are senile plaques (SPs), neurofibrillary tangles and Lewy's body (LB) deposition [106]. SPs are extracellular amyloids stored in gray matter and a normal aged brain demonstrates a moderate density of SPs. Neurofibrillary tangles (NT) represent intraneuronal aggregation of tau protein. LBs are the intraneuronal storage of alpha-synuclein and ubiquitin [106]. In addition to conventional multi-parametric MRI, MRS now represents an irreplaceable diagnostic tool that can confirm and monitor disease progression and the effects of therapies.

AD is the most common primitive brain dementia with sporadic onset. Neuropathologic features are the same as mentioned above, including the peculiar anatomic pattern of deposition of SPs and NTs within the medial temporal and hippocampal regions, in the early stages, with secondary involvement of the paralimbic regions, and entorhinal and association cortices. Morphologic evaluation in conventional 1.5 or 3 T MRI shows thinned gyri, widened sulci and enlarged ventricles. Furthermore, T2* sequences are useful to identify amyloid-related cortical microbleeds [107]. MRS may show typical patterns of decreased levels of NAA within the medial temporal lobe, hippocampal regions, parietal cortex and posterior cingulate, and increased levels of mI within the medial temporal lobes, parieto-occipital cortex and prefrontal cortex. These biomarkers (NAA and mI) may be sensitive predictors of the severity of disease and NAA/mI together with NAA/Cr in medio-occipital regions can positively relate to mini-mental-state-examination (MMSE) scores and clinical outcomes of the disease [108].

DLB is a synucleinopathy related to mutation in the alpha-synuclein gene, shared by Parkinson's disease (PD), multisystem atrophy (MSA) and REM behavior disorders (RBD), with LB intraneuronal inclusions within the substantia nigra and dorsal meso-pontine gray matter and typical loss of tegmental dopamine and basal forebrain cholinergic neurons [109]. Conventional MRI generally shows a mild to moderate frontotemporal and parietal atrophy, with hypothalamic and putaminal involvement in severe cases, and hippocampal and occipital sparing. MRS may show low NAA/Cr, Glx/Cr and Cho/Cr within the posterior cingulate gyrus without any relationship to neuropsychological performance [110].

FTD is a heterogeneous group of disorders affecting the frontal and temporal lobes, and is caused by three main mutations with three main clinical syndromes: the behavioral variant (bv-FTD), associated with personality changes; the semantic variant (s-FTD), associated with behavioral changes and altered comprehension of language; and the progressive non-fluent variant (pnf-FTD), which manifests in expressive language disorders [111]. These clinical variants show specific patterns of regional atrophy into bilateral temporal lobes without frontal involvement (s-FTD) or bilateral atrophy into frontal and temporal lobes (bv-FTD and pnf-FTD) [111]. The macroscopic signs of this spectrum are gliosis with neuronal loss and spongiosis, which cause 'knife-like' narrowing of the frontal and temporal gyri, associated with accumulation of the aggregated proteins tau, TDP-43 and FUS [112]. Conventional MRI depicts different patterns of brain atrophy and white matter damage in T2W sequences, with frequent restricted diffusion in the superior frontal gyrus, orbito-frontal gyrus and anterior temporal lobes [112]. Spectroscopic analysis shows an increased peak of mI and typical reduction of NAA and Glx peaks in the frontal regions, which differentiates FTD from AD, with a relative increase of mI/Cr and a decrease of NAA/Cr, probably located in the posterior cingulate gyrus [113].

Vascular dementia (VD) is the most common cause of dementia after AD. VD is an acquired sporadic condition, associated with acute and chronic vascular injuries such as TIA, stroke or small vessel diseases (SVD) [114]. There are many others rare monogenic disorders that cause VD, such as cerebral autosomal-dominant (CADASIL) or recessive (CARASIL) arteriopathy with subcortical infarcts and leukoencephalopathy, Fabry's disease, and pontine autosomal-dominant micro-angiopathy and leukoencephalopathy (PADMAL). The MRS patterns are very similar and typically show reduced NAA/Cr and higher Cho/Cr within frontal and parietal white and gray matter, while Herminghaus *et al* demonstrated elevated levels of mI and mI/Cr in both white and gray matter [114]. As the number of ischemic lacunes increases, the NAA peak becomes smaller and smaller [115]. Differential diagnosis between VD and AD is very difficult and MRS may help in the diagnostic work-up. In particular, VD patients show lower NAA/Cr and NAA/Cho than AD patients in subcortical frontal parietal white matter and gray matter [116].

ALS and HD are rarer causes of neurodegeneration with genetically determined secondary dementia. ALS is a sporadic or, less frequently, familial pathologic condition of progressive anterograde-retrograde degeneration of motor neurons affecting the precentral gyrus, motor cortex, brainstem and anterior horns of the spinal cord [117]. ALS is included in the FTLD spectrum and its dominant clinical phenotype is muscle weakness leading to atrophy and paralysis; dementia can occur, but rarely. The MRI appearance of ALS shows the macroscopic atrophy of precentral gyrus gray matter in T1W sequences. T2W-FLAIR can show hyperintensity of precentral gyrus subcortical white matter, the posterior limb of the internal capsule and cerebral peduncles. T2* sequences can eventually show focal hypointensity in these regions [118]. MRS can be useful to set the metabolic integrity of precentral gray matter and the other regions involved, showing reduced levels of glutamate and NAA, with relative ratios (NAA/Cr and NAA/Cho), and higher levels of mI in both the affected and unaffected motor cortex of both hemispheres [119]. In particular, high values of NAA/Cr and NAA/Cho, higher than a median value of 2.1 ppm, relate to good clinical outcomes and survival rates and they could represent biomarkers of the advanced stage of disease and effective response to drug therapies [120].

HD is an autosomal-dominant chronic hereditary syndrome caused by intersynaptic and nuclear aggregation of 'huntingtin' protein, which leads to the death of medium spiny neurons with secondary atrophy of neostriatum (NS) and globus pallidus (GP) [121]. Conventional MRI shows diffuse brain atrophy of the frontal lobes and hyperintensity of NS and GP on T2W sequences in the early stages of disease. Morphometric and tractography studies demonstrate preclinical abnormalities of hemispheric white matter and cortex [122]. MRS may show many heterogeneous patterns of several metabolites, such as Lac, Cho and Glx. In particular, several studies confirmed elevated Lac levels in the NS, GP, occipital cortex and cerebellum as a result of impaired oxidative metabolism [123]. In the medial frontal cortex, MRS can detect decreased peaks of Cho and elevated Glx/Cr, with normal levels of Glx, as results of glutamate excitotoxicity and predictable preclinical biomarkers of disease [124].

4.8 Conclusion and future perspectives

As seen in this brief chapter, *in vivo* MRS represents an integrated MRI tool that is becoming more and more irreplaceable in the diagnostic work-up of many neurological disorders, providing information about metabolic changes that are useful to monitor the progression, regression and drug-response of disease. This chapter described the most common spectroscopic profiles of adult diseases and indicated some pediatric congenital neurologic disorders, such as FCD, HIE and other inherited metabolic conditions, giving some target-points for correct diagnostic assessment.

Critical issues for the correct and reproducible spectroscopic examination and quality of spectra are both the experience and technical skills of the reading operators, and the quality of the MRI scanner system and MRS software. Future aims are the increasing integration and standardization of *in vivo* MRS techniques and the development of automated methods of analysis, taking advantage of artificial intelligence technology (AIT) such as deep learning algorithms and big data analysis.

References

[1] Proctor W G and Yu F C 1950 The dependence of nuclear magnetic resonance frequency upon chemical compound *Phys. Rev.* **70** 717

[2] Frahm J 1987 Localized proton spectroscopy using stimulated echoes *J. Magn. Reson.* **72** 502–8

[3] Benuck M and D'Adamo J A 1968 Acetyl transport mechanisms. Metabolism of N-acetyl-L-aspartic acid in the non-nervous tissues of the rat *Biochim. Biophys. Acta* **152** 611–8

[4] Urenjak J *et al* 1992 Specific expression of N-acetylaspartate in neurons, oligodendrocyte-type-2 astrocyte progenitors, and immature oligodendrocytes *in vitro J. Neurochem.* **59** 55–61

[5] Bertholdo D, Watcharakorn A and Castillo M 2013 Brain proton magnetic resonance spectroscopy: introduction and overview *Neuroimaging Clin. N. Am.* **23** 359–80

[6] Bruhn H *et al* 1989 Noninvasive differentiation of tumors with use of localized H-1 MR spectroscopy *in vivo*: initial experience in patients with cerebral tumors *Radiology* **172** 541–8

[7] Miller S P 2007 Newborn brain injury: looking back to the fetus *Ann. Neurol.* **61** 285–7

[8] Weeke L C *et al* 2018 A novel magnetic resonance imaging score predicts neurodevelopmental outcome after perinatal asphyxia and therapeutic hypothermia *J. Pediatr.* **192** 33–40

[9] Chao C P, Zaleski C G and Patton A C 2006 Neonatal hypoxic-ischemic encephalopathy: multimodality imaging findings *Radiographics* **26** S159–72

[10] Barkovich A J *et al* 2006 MR imaging, MR spectroscopy, and diffusion tensor imaging of sequential studies in neonates with encephalopathy *AJNR Am. J. Neuroradiol.* **27** 533–47

[11] Shu S K *et al* 1997 Prognostic value of 1-H ERM in perinatal CNS insults *Pediatr. Neurol.* **17** 309–18

[12] Huang B Y and Castillo M 2008 Hypoxic–ischemic brain injury: imaging findings from birth to adulthood *Radiographics* **28** 417–39

[13] Barkovich A J *et al* 1999 Proton MR spectroscopy for the evaluation of brain injury in asphyxiated, term neonates *AJNR Am. J. Neuroradiol.* **20** 1399–405

[14] Ross B D, Ernest T and Kries R 1995 Proton magnetic resonance spectroscopy in hypoxic–ischemic disorders *MRI of the Central Nervous System in Infants and Children* ed M Bax and E N Faerber (London: MacKeith) pp 279–306

[15] Danielsen E R and Ross B 1999 *Magnetic Resonance Spectroscopy Diagnosis of Neurological Diseases* (New York: Marcel Dekker) pp 147–85

[16] Zarifi M K *et al* 2002 Prediction of adverse outcome with cerebral lactate level and apparent diffusion coefficient in infants with perinatal asphyxia *Radiology* **225** 859–70

[17] Horská A and Barker P B 2010 Imaging of brain tumors: MR spectroscopy and metabolic imaging *Neuroimaging Clin. N. Am.* **20** 293–310

[18] Tennant D A, Durán R V and Gottlieb E 2010 Targeting metabolic transformation for cancer therapy *Nat. Rev. Cancer* **10** 267–77

[19] Warburg O 1956 On the origin of cancer cells *Science* **123** 309–14

[20] Chiche J, Ilc K, Laferrière J, Trottier E, Dayan F, Mazure N M, Brahimi-Horn M C and Pouysségur J 2009 Hypoxia-inducible carbonic anhydrase IX and XII promote tumor cell growth by counteracting acidosis through the regulation of the intracellular pH *Cancer Res.* **69** 358–68

[21] Papandreou I, Cairns R A, Fontana L, Lim A L and Denko N C 2006 HIF-1 mediates adaptation to hypoxia by actively downregulating mitochondrial oxygen consumption *Cell Metab.* **3** 187–97

[22] Snell K 1984 Enzymes of serine metabolism in normal developing and neoplastic rat tissues *Adv. Enzyme Regul.* **22** 325–400

[23] Maudsley A A, Gupta R K, Stoyanova R, Parra N A, Roy B, Sheriff S, Hussain N and Behari S 2014 Mapping of glycine distributions in gliomas *AJNR Am. J. Neuroradiol.* **35** S31–6

[24] Hattingen E, Raab P, Franz K, Zanella F E, Lanfermann H and Pilatus U 2008 Myo-inositol: a marker of reactive astrogliosis in glial tumors? *NMR Biomed.* **21** 233–41

[25] Hattingen E, Lanfermann H, Quick J, Franz K, Zanella F E and Pilatus U 2009 ^{1}H MR spectroscopic imaging with short and long echo time to discriminate glycine in glial tumours *MAGMA* **22** 33–41

[26] Herminghaus S, Pilatus U, Möller-Hartmann W, Raab P, Lanfermann H, Schlote W and Zanella F E 2002 Increased choline levels coincide with enhanced proliferative activity of human neuroepithelial brain tumors *NMR Biomed.* **15** 385–92

[27] Kennedy E P 1957 Metabolism of lipids *Annu. Rev. Biochem.* **26** 119–48

[28] Glunde K, Shah T, Winnard P T Jr, Raman V, Takagi T, Vesuna F, Artemov D and Bhujwalla Z M 2008 Hypoxia regulates choline kinase expression through hypoxia-inducible factor-1 alpha signaling in a human prostate cancer model *Cancer Res.* **68** 172–80

[29] Hattingen E, Bähr O, Rieger J, Blasel S, Steinbach J and Pilatus U 2013 Phospholipid metabolites in recurrent glioblastoma: *in vivo* markers detect different tumor phenotypes before and under antiangiogenic therapy *PLoS One* **8** e56439

[30] Zoula S, Herigault G, Ziegler A, Farion R, Decorps M and Remy C 2003 Correlation between the occurrence of ^{1}H-MRS lipid signal, necrosis and lipid droplets during C6 rat glioma development *NMR Biomed.* **16** 199

[31] Cha S 2006 Update on brain tumor imaging: from anatomy to physiology *AJNR Am. J. Neuroradiol.* **27** 475

[32] Stadlbauer A, Moser E, Gruber S, Buslei R, Nimsky C, Fahlbusch R and Ganslandt O 2004 Improved delineation of brain tumors: an automated method for segmentation based on pathologic changes of ^{1}H-MRSI metabolites in gliomas *Neuroimage* **23** 454

[33] Martínez-Bisbal M C *et al* 2015 *Anal. Bioanal. Chem.* **407** 6771

[34] Ziegler A, von Kienlin M, Decorps M and Remy C 2001 High glycolytic activity in rat glioma demonstrated *in vivo* by correlation peak ^{1}H magnetic resonance imaging *Cancer Res.* **61** 5595

[35] Steinberg J D and Velan S S 2012 Measuring glucose concentrations in the rat brain using echo-time-averaged point resolved spectroscopy at 7 tesla *Magn. Reson. Med.* **70** 301–8

[36] Mörén L *et al* 2015 Metabolomic screening of tumor tissue and serum in glioma patients reveals diagnostic and prognostic information *Metabolites* **5** 502–20
[37] Porto L, Kieslich M, Franz K, Lehrbecher T, Pilatus U and Hattingen E 2010 Proton magnetic resonance spectroscopic imaging in pediatric low-grade gliomas *Brain Tumor Pathol.* **27** 65–70
[38] Castillo M, Smith J K and Kwock L 2000 Correlation of myo-inositol levels and grading of cerebral astrocytomas *AJNR Am. J. Neuroradiol.* **21** 1645–9
[39] Hattingen E, Delic O, Franz K, Pilatus U, Raab P, Lanfermann H and Gerlach R 2010 ^{1}H MRSI and progression-free survival in patients with WHO grades II and III gliomas *Neurol. Res.* **32** 593–602
[40] Stadlbauer A, Nimsky C, Buslei R, Pinker K, Gruber S, Hammen T, Buchfelder M and Ganslandt O 2007 Proton magnetic resonance spectroscopic imaging in the border zone of gliomas: correlation of metabolic and histological changes at low tumor infiltration—initial results *Invest. Radiol.* **42** 218–23
[41] Harting I, Hartmann M, Jost G, Sommer C, Ahmadi R, Heiland S and Sartor K 2003 Differentiating primary central nervous system lymphoma from glioma in humans using localised proton magnetic resonance spectroscopy *Neurosci. Lett.* **342** 163–6
[42] Poptani H, Gupta R K, Roy R, Pandey R, Jain V K and Chhabra D K 1995 Characterization of intracranial mass lesions with *in vivo* proton MR spectroscopy *AJNR Am. J. Neuroradiol.* **16** 1593–603
[43] Kovanlikaya A, Panigrahy A, Krieger M D, Gonzalez-Gomez I, Ghugre N, McComb J G, Gilles F H, Nelson M D and Blüml S 2005 Untreated pediatric primitive neuroectodermal tumor *in vivo*: quantitation of taurine with MR spectroscopy *Radiology* **236** 1020–5
[44] Di Costanzo A *et al* 2008 Proton MR spectroscopy of cerebral gliomas at 3 T: spatial heterogeneity, tumour grade and extent *Eur. Radiol.* **18** 1727–35
[45] Kreis R 2004 Issues of spectral quality in clinical ^{1}H-magnetic resonance spectroscopy and a gallery of artifacts *NMR Biomed.* **17** 361–81
[46] Cendes F *et al* 1997 Proton magnetic resonance spectroscopic imaging for discrimination of absence and complex partial seizures *Ann. Neurol.* **41** 74–81
[47] Parikh S *et al* 2008 Metabolic testing in the pediatric epilepsy unit *Pediatr. Neurol.* **38** 191–5
[48] Canafoglia L *et al* 2001 Epileptic phenotypes associated with mitochondrial disorders *Neurology* **56** 1340–6
[49] Cristina Bianchi M *et al* 2003 Proton MR spectroscopy of mitochondrial diseases: analysis of brain metabolic abnormalities and their possible diagnostic relevance *AJNR Am. J. Neuroradiol.* **24** 1958–66
[50] Stromberger C, Bodamer O A and Stockler-Ipsiroglu S 2003 Clinical characteristics and diagnostic clues in inborn errors of creatine metabolism *J. Inherit. Metab. Dis.* **26** 299–308
[51] Palmini A *et al* 1995 Intrinsic epileptogenicity of human dysplastic cortex as suggested by corticography and surgical results *Ann. Neurol.* **37** 476–87
[52] Mueller S G *et al* 2005 Metabolic characteristics of cortical malformations causing epilepsy *J. Neurol.* **252** 1082–92
[53] Tschampa H J *et al* Proton magnetic resonance spectroscopy in focal cortical dysplasia at 3 T seizure *Eur. J. Epilepsy* **32** 23–9
[54] Negendank W G *et al* 1996 Proton magnetic resonance spectroscopy in patients with glial tumors: a multicenter study *J. Neurosurg.* **84** 449–58

[55] Cendes F *et al* 1997 Proton magnetic resonance spectroscopic imaging and magnetic resonance imaging volumetry in the lateralization of temporal lobe epilepsy: a series of 100 patients *Ann. Neurol.* **42** 737–46

[56] Kuzniecky R *et al* 1998 Relative utility of ^{1}H spectroscopic imaging and hippocampal volumetry in the lateralization of mesial temporal lobe epilepsy *Neurology* **51** 66–71

[57] Campos B *et al* 2010 Proton MRS may predict AED response in patients with TLE *Epilepsia* **51** 783–8

[58] Peruzzotti-Jametti L, Donega M, Giusto E, Mallucci G, Marchetti B and Pluchino S 2014 The role of the immune system in central nervous system plasticity after acute injury *Neuroscience* **283** 210–21

[59] Jacobs A H and Tavitian B 2012 Noninvasive molecular imaging of neuroinflammation *J. Cereb. Blood Flow Metab.* **32** 1393–415

[60] Anlar O 2009 Treatment of multiple sclerosis *CNS Neurol. Disord. Drug Targets* **8** 167–74

[61] Neumann H 2003 Molecular mechanisms of axonal damage in inflammatory central nervous system diseases *Curr. Opin. Neurol.* **16** 267–73

[62] Yamout B I and Alroughani R 2018 Multiple sclerosis *Semin. Neurol.* **38** 212–25

[63] De Stefano N *et al* 2001 Evidence of axonal damage in the early stages of multiple sclerosis and its relevance to disability *Arch. Neurol.* **58** 65–70

[64] Bitsch A *et al* 1999 Inflammatory CNS demyelination: histopathologic correlation with *in vivo* quantitative proton MR spectroscopy *AJNR Am. J. Neuroradiol.* **20** 1619–27

[65] De Stefano N and Filippi M 2007 MR spectroscopy in multiple sclerosis *J. Neuroimaging* **17** 31S–5

[66] Mader I *et al* 2001 Proton MR spectroscopy with metabolite-nulling reveals elevated macromolecules in acute multiple sclerosis *Brain* **124** 953–61

[67] Kapeller P *et al* 2001 Preliminary evidence for neuronal damage in cortical grey matter and normal appearing white matter in short duration relapsing–remitting multiple sclerosis: a quantitative MR spectroscopic imaging study *J. Neurol.* **248** 131–8

[68] Chard D T *et al* 2002 Brain metabolite changes in cortical grey and normal-appearing white matter in clinically early relapsing–remitting multiple sclerosis *Brain* **125** 2342–52

[69] Ben Sira L, Miller E, Artzi M, Fattal-Valevski A, Constantini S and Ben Bashat D 2010 ^{1}H-MRS for the diagnosis of acute disseminated encephalomyelitis: insight into the acute-disease stage *Pediatr. Radiol.* **40** 106–13

[70] Cianfoni A, Niku S and Imbesi S G 2007 Metabolite findings in tumefactive demyelinating lesions utilizing short echo time proton magnetic resonance spectroscopy *Am. J. Neuroradiol.* **28** 272–7

[71] Kastrup O, Wanke I and Maschke M 2008 Neuroimaging of infections of the central nervous system *Semin. Neurol.* **28** 511–22

[72] Brook I 2017 Microbiology and treatment of brain abscess *J. Clin. Neurosci.* **38** 8–12

[73] Haimes A B *et al* 1989 MR imaging of brain abscesses *AJR Am. J. Roentgenol.* **152** 1073–85

[74] Shukla-Dave A *et al* 2001 Prospective evaluation of *in vivo* proton MR spectroscopy in differentiation of similar appearing intracranial cystic lesions *Magn. Reson. Imaging* **19** 103–10

[75] Garg M *et al* 2004 Brain abscesses: etiologic categorization with *in vivo* proton MR spectroscopy *Radiology* **230** 519

[76] Chiang I C, Hsieh T J, Chiu M L, Liu G C, Kuo Y T and Lin W C 2009 Distinction between pyogenic brain abscess and necrotic brain tumour using 3-tesla MR spectroscopy, diffusion and perfusion imaging *Br. J. Radiol.* **82** 813–20

[77] Be N A, Kim K S, Bishai W R and Jain S K 2009 Pathogenesis of central nervous system tuberculosis *Curr. Mol. Med.* **9** 94–9

[78] Morgado C and Ruivo N 2005 Imaging meningo-encephalic tuberculosis *Eur. J. Radiol.* **55** 188–92

[79] Poptani H, Kaartinen J, Gupta R K, Niemitz M, Hiltunen Y and Kauppinen R A 1999 Diagnostic assessment of brain tumours and nonneoplastic brain disorders *in vivo* using proton nuclear magnetic resonance spectroscopy and artificial neural networks *J. Cancer Res. Clin. Oncol.* **125** 343–9

[80] Todeschi J, Gubian A, Wirth T, Coca H A, Proust F and Cebula H 2018 Multimodal management of severe herpes simplex virus encephalitis: a case report and literature review *Neurochirurgie* **64** 183–9

[81] Takanashi J, Sugita K, Ishii M, Aoyagi M and Niimi H 1997 Longitudinal MR imaging and proton MR spectroscopy in herpes simplex encephalitis *J. Neurol. Sci.* **149** 99–102

[82] Yamaguchi Y, Igari R, Tanji H and Kato T 2015 HIV encephalopathy as an initial manifestation of AIDS *Intern. Med.* **54** 2423

[83] Chang L *et al* 1999 Highly active antiretroviral therapy reverses brain metabolite abnormalities in mild HIV dementia *Neurology* **53** 782–9

[84] Simone I L *et al* 1998 Localised ^{1}H-MR spectroscopy for metabolic characterisation of diffuse and focal brain lesions in patients infected with HIV *J. Neurol. Neurosurg. Psychiatry* **64** 516–23

[85] Zacharia T T, Law M, Naidich T P and Leeds N E 2008 Central nervous system lymphoma characterization by diffusion-weighted imaging and MR spectroscopy *J. Neuroimaging* **18** 411–7

[86] Rovira A, Alonso J and Cordoba J 2008 MR imaging findings in hepatic encephalopathy *AJNR Am. J. Neuroradiol.* **29** 1612e21

[87] Haussinger D and Schliess F 2005 Astrocyte swelling and protein tyrosine nitration in hepatic encephalopathy *Neurochem. Int.* **47** 64–70

[88] Sharma P, Eesa M and Scott J N 2009 Toxic and acquired metabolic encephalopathies: MRI appearance *AJR Am. J. Roentgenol.* **193** 879e86

[89] Naegele T *et al* 2000 MR imaging and ^{1}H spectroscopy of brain metabolites in hepatic encephalopathy: time-course of renormalization after liver transplantation *Radiology* **216** 683–91

[90] Malouf R and Brust J C 1985 Hypoglycemia: causes, neurological manifestations, and outcome *Ann. Neurol.* **17** 421e30

[91] Hegde A N *et al* 2011 Differential diagnosis for bilateral abnormalities of the basal ganglia and thalamus *Radiographics* **31** 5e30

[92] Fujioka M *et al* 1997 Specific changes in human brain after hypoglycemic injury *Stroke* **28** 584e7

[93] Aoki T *et al* 2004 Reversible hyperintensity lesion on diffusion-weighted MRI in hypoglycemic coma *Neurology* **63** 392e3

[94] Zuccoli G and Pipitone N 2009 Neuroimaging findings in acute Wernicke's encephalopathy: review of the literature *AJR Am. J. Roentgenol.* **192** 501e8

[95] Harper C and Butterworth R 1997 Nutritional and metabolic disorders *Greenfield's Neuropathology* vol 1 6th edn ed D I Graham and P L Lantos (London: Hodder Arnold) p 601e52

[96] Zuccoli G *et al* 2009 MR imaging findings in 56 patients with Wernicke encephalopathy: nonalcoholics may differ from alcoholics *AJNR Am. J. Neuroradiol.* **30** 171e6

[97] Murata T, Fujito T, Kimura H, Omori M, Itoh H and Wada Y 2001 Serial MRI and ^{1}H-MRS of Wernicke's encephalopathy: report of a case with remarkable cerebellar lesions on MRI *Psychiatry Res.* **108** 49–55

[98] Mascalchi M, Belli G, Guerrini L, Nistri M, Del Seppia I and Villari N 2002 Proton MR spectroscopy of Wernicke encephalopathy *AJNR Am. J. Neuroradiol.* **23** 1803–6

[99] Chuang D T, Chuang J L and Wynn R M 2006 Lessons from genetic disorders of branched-chain amino acid metabolism *J. Nutr.* **136** 243S–9

[100] Jan W *et al* 2003 *Neuroradiology* **45** 393

[101] Möller H E *et al* 2011 Brain imaging and proton magnetic resonance spectroscopy in patients with phenylketonuria *Pediatrics* **112** 1580–3

[102] Schulze A 2003 Creatine deficiency syndromes *Mol. Cell. Biochem.* **244** 143–50

[103] Rosewich H *et al* 2016 *J. Inherit. Metab. Dis.* **39** 869

[104] Dinopoulos A *et al* 2005 Brain MRI and proton MRS findings in infants and children with respiratory chain defects *Neuropediatrics* **36** 290–301

[105] Charidimou A and Viswanathan A 2016 Multiple neuropathologies and dementia in the aging brain: a key role for cerebrovascular disease? *Alzheimer's Dement.* **2** 281–2

[106] Savva G M *et al* 2009 Age neuropathology, and dementia *N. Engl. J. Med.* **360** 2302–9

[107] Chetelat G and Baron J C 2003 Early diagnosis of Alzheimer's disease: contribution of structural neuroimaging *Neuroimage* **18** 525–41

[108] Waldman A D and Rai G S 2003 The relationship between cognitive impairment and *in vivo* metabolite ratios in patients with clinical Alzheimer's disease and vascular dementia: a proton magnetic resonance spectroscopy study *Neuroradiology* **45** 507–12

[109] Tartaglia M C, Rosen H J and Miller B L 2011 Neuroimaging in dementia *Neurotherapeutics* **8** 82–92

[110] Molina J A *et al* 2002 Proton magnetic resonance spectroscopy in dementia with Lewy bodies *Eur. Neurol.* **48** 158–63

[111] Woollacott I O and Rohrer J D 2016 The clinical spectrum of sporadic and familial forms of frontotemporal dementia *J. Neurochem.* **138** 6–31

[112] Bang J, Spina S and Miller B L 2015 Non-Alzheimer's dementia 1: frontotemporal dementia *Lancet* **386** 1672–82

[113] Mihara M, Hattori N, Abe K, Sakoda S and Sawada T 2006 Magnetic resonance spectroscopic study of Alzheimer's disease and frontotemporal dementia/Pick complex *Neuroreport* **17** 413–6

[114] Herminghaus S *et al* 2003 Brain metabolism in Alzheimer disease and vascular dementia assessed by *in vivo* proton magnetic resonance spectroscopy *Psychiatry Res.* **123** 183–90

[115] Schuff N *et al* 2003 Different patterns of N-acetylaspartate loss in subcorticalischemic vascular dementia and AD *Neurology* **61** 358–64

[116] MacKay S, Meyerhoff D J, Constans J M, Norman D, Fein G and Weiner M W 1996 Regional gray and white matter metabolite differences in subjects with AD, with subcortical ischemic vascular dementia, and elderly controls with ^{1}H magnetic resonance spectroscopic imaging *Arch. Neurol.* **53** 167–74

[117] Azuma Y, Mizuta I, Tokuda T and Mizuno T 2018 Amyotrophic lateral sclerosis model *Drosophila Models for Human Diseases. Advances in Experimental Medicine and Biology* vol 1076 ed M Yamaguchi (Singapore: Springer)

[118] Menke R A L *et al* 2014 Widespread grey matter pathology dominates the longitudinal cerebral MRI and clinical landscape of amyotrophic lateral sclerosis *Brain* **137** 2546–55

[119] Wang Y, Li X, Chen W, Wang Z, Xu Y, Luo J, Lin H and Sun G 2017 Detecting neuronal dysfunction of hand motor cortex in ALS: a MRSI study *Somatosens. Mot. Res.* **34** 15–20

[120] Kalra S, Tai P, Genge A and Arnold D L 2006 Rapid improvement in corticalneuronal integrity in amyotrophic lateral sclerosis detected by proton magnetic resonance spectroscopic imaging *J. Neurol.* **253** 1060–3

[121] Gil J M and Rego A C 2008 Mechanisms of neurodegeneration in Huntington's disease *Eur. J. Neurosci.* **27** 2803–20

[122] Paulsen J S *et al* 2014 Prediction of manifest Huntington's disease with clinical and imaging measures: a prospective observational study *Lancet Neurol.* **13** 1193–201

[123] Jenkins B G, Koroshetz W J, Beal M F and Rosen B R 1993 Evidence for impairment of energy metabolism *in vivo* in Huntington's disease using localized ^{1}H NMR spectroscopy *Neurology* **43** 2689–95

[124] Taylor-Robinson S D *et al* 1996 Proton magnetic resonance spectroscopy in Huntington's disease: evidence in favour of the glutamate excitotoxic theory *Mov. Disord.* **11** 167–73

IOP Publishing

Neurological Disorders and Imaging Physics, Volume 1
Application of multiple sclerosis
Luca Saba and Jasjit S Suri

Chapter 5

High field MR and neurological disorders

James T Grist, Frank Riemer, Tomasz Matys, Rhys Slough and Fulvio Zaccagna

Magnetic resonance imaging (MRI) is commonly described in terms of the strength of the main magnetic field (B_0). 'High field MR' refers to the most commonly used clinical field strengths, 1.5–3.0 Tesla (T). However, the push towards higher fields led to whole-body systems beyond 3 T, called 'very high' (4.7–7.0 T) and 'ultra-high' (>7 T) field systems. The latter systems are increasingly used for research, particularly in neuro-imaging, as high spatial resolutions (<1 mm isotropic) are achievable in relatively short scan times, unleashing the possibility of assessing brain microstructure on a very fine scale. Recently, the first brain MRI scan at 10.5 T was acquired at the Center for Magnetic Resonance Research—University of Minnesota as part of the Human Connectome Project. However, despite the interest on the research side, very high and ultra-high field strength magnets are still far from being in routine clinical use.

In this chapter we will review the rationale behind high field MRI, and the challenges, applications and future developments. Although according to the definition of high field MRI the magnet strength we will refer to is 3 T, we would like to highlight that most of the considerations are valid for higher field strengths as well.

5.1 The rationale for high field MRI

The rationale for using high field MRI can be either clinical or technical, although the latter is closely related to the former. Despite the key relevance of MRI in the diagnosis and monitoring of MS, conventional imaging has many shortcomings. The signal changes visualised on T_1WI, T_2WI and FLAIR images in patients with suspected multiple sclerosis are non-specific, and can indicate inflammation, demyelination, ischaemia, oedema or gliosis among others. Moreover, conventional imaging lacks the capacity of reliably assessing the degree of injury and accurately identifying and quantifying the lesion burden (i.e. at 1.5 T cortical lesions are hard to depict) [1].

doi:10.1088/2053-2563/ab1fdcch5

When it comes to the technical push, there are a number of advantages to acquiring MR imaging and spectroscopy at higher field strengths, primarily due to the increased polarisation of nuclear magnetic resonance active nuclei with higher field strength:

$$\text{Polarisation} = \tanh\left(\frac{h\gamma B_0}{2\pi k_b T}\right), \tag{5.1}$$

where h is Plank's constant (m^2 kg s^{-1}), γ is the gyromagnetic ratio (MHz T^{-1}), B_0 is the main field strength (T), k_b is Boltzmann's constant (m^2 kg s^{-2} K^{-1}) and T is the temperature of the system (K) (assumed body temperature).

The increase in polarisation leads to a subsequent increase in the MRI signal available during acquisitions, which can be leveraged in different ways. Primarily, this can be used to increase the imaging spatial resolution in sequences that commonly are signal-to-noise ratio (SNR) limited at 1.5 T (for example, double inversion recovery fast spin echo, where multiple inversion recovery pulses used to null cerebrospinal fluid and white matter cause a large decrease in the total available signal prior to acquisition). Second, the increase in SNR can be used to accelerate acquisitions, for example in magnetic resonance spectroscopy (MRS) where a large number of averages are required to obtain signal from low concentration metabolites.

However, the benefits of moving to higher field strengths are not just found in an increased SNR, with also an increased spectroscopic frequency dispersion proportional to field strength:

$$f = \gamma\sigma, \tag{5.2}$$

where f is the resonant frequency of a metabolite (Hz), γ is as above and σ (ppm) is the chemical shift relative to tetramethylsilane (an organosilicon compound used as reference from which chemical shifts are measured in MRS). Moving from 1.5 T to 3 T enables better discrimination between metabolites such as creatine and choline, as well as a general increase in SNR at low echo times [2].

5.2 Challenges, safety issues and limitations

There are a number of challenges that arise due to the increase in field strength, primarily concerning safety and potential longer acquisitions times. Due to the increasing field strength, higher radiofrequency (RF) energy is required to excite spins in the body, leading to larger energy deposition throughout imaging. Indeed, the increase in specific absorption rate (SAR) is proportional to the squared increase in field strength, and so moving from 1.5 T to 3.0 T can bring significant amplification in energy deposition for equivalent acquisitions. This surge in specific absorption rate is particularly challenging for sequences such as magnetisation transfer (MT) imaging, where radiofrequency pulses with high energy deposition are required to obtain magnetisation transfer contrast.

Energy deposition is carefully monitored in clinical systems, with changes to RF pulse lengths, sequence repetition time (TR) and excitation flip angle used to ensure energy deposition is kept within accepted limits.

Furthermore, the resonant frequency of nuclei increases with field strength (as shown in equation (5.3)). This increase in field strength leads to longer RF wavelengths being required to excite spins, which causes an inhomogeneous distribution of RF across the field of view, and apparent alterations in image contrast (this is termed 'transmit B1 inhomogeneity'):

$$f = \gamma B_0, \tag{5.3}$$

where f is the resonant frequency of nuclei (Hz), and γ and B_0 are as above. Methods for the correction of B1 inhomogeneity range from increasing the number of transmit channels in a coil to acquiring a B1 map and mathematically correcting images after acquisition.

Finally, moving between 1.5 T and 3 T can lead to changes in the longitudinal relaxation time of nuclei. Generally, a lengthening of T1 is observed between 1.5 T and 3.0 T, leading to longer delays between each RF excitation to allow for complete signal relaxation. This, in turn, leads to longer scan times for techniques that require inversion pulses to null tissues, for example T2 FLAIR or double inversion recovery.

5.3 High field applications

The diverse and copious advantages of high field MRI can be potentially exploited for imaging several neurological conditions. The use of non-invasive imaging revolutionised the management of multiple sclerosis. Indeed, due to a combination of the sheer number of afflicted patients and a need for improved non-invasive imaging techniques, multiple sclerosis has been one of the earliest applications to be explored using high field MRI [3]. In the quest for earlier detection, improved patients classification, follow-up assessment and quantification, high field MRI was evaluated as a novel tool to assess lesion localisation and disease burden.

The magnetic field strength significantly influences the detection of small, millimetric, lesions as first demonstrated by Keiper [4] comparing a 1.5 T and a 4 T system. In his seminal paper, Keiper *et al* demonstrated a 45% increase in lesion detection with the stronger magnet on T_2WI sequences. Several papers confirmed the capability of 3 T magnets to detect a higher number of lesions using T_2WI, FLAIR and T_1WI post (30, 32) with subsequent worse radiological classification resulting from the increased lesion burden [5]. However, interestingly, the increase in the lesion load does not directly translate into a re-classification of patients nor into earlier diagnosis when considering clinical features [6, 7].

5.3.1 Faster acquisition strategies

The manifold increase in SNR provided by higher field magnets can be harnessed for either improving the spatial and contrast resolution or for shortening the acquisition time. In an age and era of continuous increase in the number of prescribed radiological examinations, characterised by the rocketing numbers of performed

MRIs, a decrease in scan time can be beneficial to increase the number of patients that can benefit from an MRI in a busy clinical practice. Many protocols have been proposed to accelerate the scan time, including fast spin echo techniques, variable flip angle refocusing, half-Fourier acquisition, and more advanced and sophisticated parallel imaging. The general aim is to reduce the scan time maintaining a high enough quality to be able to achieve a comparable lesion assessment and detection to 1.5 T. With this aim in mind, different research groups proposed whole brain protocols obtainable in less than 5 min [3, 8]. In our institution we have developed a 3D acquisition protocol that allows for T_1WI, T_2WI and FLAIR to be obtained in less than 15 min using a combination of acceleration in the slice and phase encoding directions, as well as reduced field of view imaging. Despite being more than two times faster than the previous standard protocol for multiple sclerosis assessment, this faster protocol allows for an increase in the conspicuity of both white matter and grey matter lesions, particularly in the brain stem, with a potential sensible advantage for the neuroradiologist reporting on the scans and remarkable benefits for patients (figure 5.1). Moreover, the availability of volumetric sequences is a remarkable advantage for surgical planning. Indeed, intended neuro-surgical navigation requires high resolution, isotropic sequences to precisely locate anatomical structures. Albeit this is usually performed using T_1WI post gadolinium administration, the information added by the availability of T_2WI and FLAIR in the surgical theatre can be invaluable. In glioma surgery, for example, FLAIR images facilitate the assessment of the extension of the peri-tumoral region of signal change potential.

5.3.2 Double inversion recovery

In addition to the improvement in conventional sequences, the introduction of magnets capable of higher field strength opened up the possibility of using novel

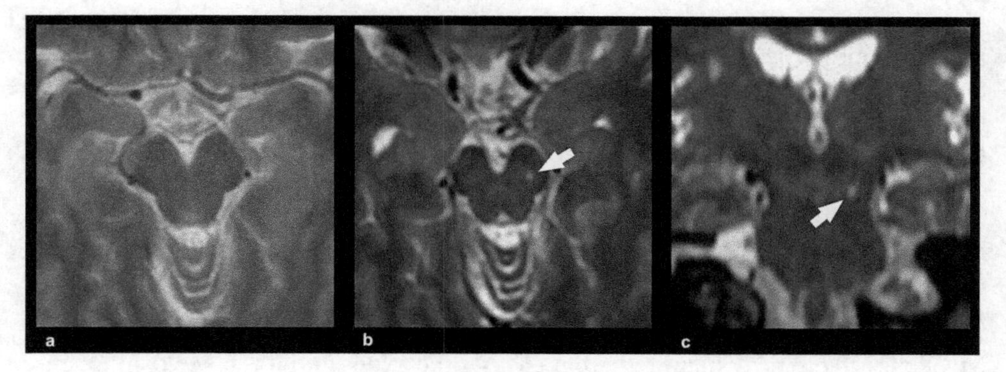

Figure 5.1. A patient with multiple sclerosis scanned with a conventional brain MRI protocol and our 'faster' 3D acquisition protocol. (a) T2 weighted image obtained as a clinical standard with a slice thickness of 6 mm. (b) T2 weighted image obtained with a isotropic volumetric acquisition (slice thickness 2 mm). (c) The coronal reformat obtained from (b). The millimetric lesion in the left cerebral peduncle is difficult to appreciate in the conventional T2 weighed image and could have been missed without careful study. In contrast, the lesion is far more evident in the volumetric T2 weighted image and is visible on multiple slices.

pulse sequences. One such sequence that has gained particular interest for its potential applications in multiple sclerosis has been double inversion recovery (DIR). This sequence utilises two simultaneous inversion pulses to suppress signals from the cerebrospinal fluid and normal white matter, improving the delineation between white matter and grey matter [9]. Although first devised in the 1990s and initially performed on 1.5 T magnets, technical limitations jeopardised its use due to poor resolution and the presence of artifacts [10]. Only with the introduction and spread of 3 T magnets has this sequence become feasible with adequate resolution.

DIR is able to improve the detection of cortical lesions when compared with 1.5 T magnets, particularly in challenging anatomical locations, such as the posterior fossa, with the capability of showing up to twice the number of lesions in the cortex when performed with 3D high resolution sequences [11]. The posterior fossa is of particular interest considering the clinical importance yielded by the infratentorial lesion load at baseline, when it comes to predicting long term disability in patients with a *de novo* diagnosis of multiple sclerosis [11]. The increase in detection and quantification of lesion burden with DIR is, as expected, related to the stronger field that allowed for higher SNR and spatial resolution. Thus, higher fields will further increase the capability of this sequence to detect grey matter lesions and quantify the lesion burden. Indeed, preliminary results with 7 T magnets have demonstrated better visualisation and detection of multiple sclerosis lesions in the cortex with the added capability of characterising their location in analogy to the histopathological typing [12–14].

5.4 Quantitative techniques

In the past 25 years, the number of available treatment strategies for multiple sclerosis have continuously increased, with a plethora of monoclonal antibodies being tested and approved, thanks to their efficacy. However, new and more aggressive therapies also yield significant risks, thus monitoring and assessment of treatment response and safety have become of paramount importance [15]. MRI plays a major role in this sense, however, conventional morphological evaluation and lesion burden quantification lack the reproducibility and the quantitative nature that would be beneficial for an imaging biomarker. Several quantitative MRI techniques have benefitted from the introduction of magnets with a field strength >1.5 T, sparking interest as potential tools for therapy assessment. Among others, T1 and T2 mapping, proton spectroscopy, diffusion imaging, magnetisation transfer imaging and functional MRI have been extensively applied in multiple sclerosis.

5.4.1 T1 and T2 mapping

Myelin is a biological membrane that encases the axons and it is a key component of the central nervous system, due to its multiple roles. Due to the obvious shielding of the conduction of the electrical impulse, myelin supplies energetic metabolites, such as lactate, and contributes to learning [16]. Therefore, if its integrity is compromised, brain functions are going to be affected. Multiple sclerosis is characterised by myelin loss and, thus, promoting remyelination can be an effective therapeutic strategy.

In harmony with this novel potential therapeutic strategy, a non-invasive assessment of myelin status has been long sought.

The T1W contrast of adult grey matter has been attributed to the cholesterol content of myelin, since a seminal paper by Koenig demonstrated that the signal obtained by phantoms built with different percentages of lipids and water mimicking the *in vivo* signal of the human brain [17]. Thus, exploiting the differences in T1W signal has been proposed as a potential way to look into myelin content. Moreover, lost myelin is replaced by free water, inflammatory cells and different proteins, also resulting in significant changes of the T2 properties of the tissue and, thus, changes in the T2W signal. However, despite the fact that the interpretation of signal changes is routine clinical practice, the intensity of the signal itself is due to underlying biological properties that are often unknown, or only partially exploited, and to several cofounding factors, including acquisition parameters, receiver coil geometry and sensitivity profile, to list just a few [18]. Therefore, the direct comparison of signal changes based on signal intensities is jeopardised by the inconsistency in acquisition, leading to the need to use more reliable and quantitative sequences for comparison across patients, different time points or different scanners. T1 (and T2) maps can address this issue, thanks to the capability of disentangling the effect of other signal components through direct calculation of the proton density and the spin relaxation times, resulting in a more direct link between the signal and the structural changes in the brain parenchyma [18]. Moreover, as the signal is derived from the tissues rather than external cofounding factors, the use of quantitative maps allows for comparisons between patients and scans obtained at different time points and with different scanners.

Similarly, it is possible to obtain T2W maps that can exploit differences in signal decay between different tissues such as, for example, between grey and white matter regions. By acquiring multiple echoes it is possible to separate tissues with different water components. In the brain, the component with the shortest relaxation time is thought to be myelin with the signal coming from the water trapped between the myelin sheaths [19]. This component has been termed the myelin water fraction (MWF) and has been extensively explored as a surrogate marker of myelin integrity. A significant reduction in the myelin water fraction has been demonstrated in multiple sclerosis lesions, which is macroscopically evident in conventional MRI, but also in normal-appearing parenchyma when compared to healthy volunteers [20]. However, Tozer *et al* compared T2 relaxation to the magnetisation transfer ratio (MTR), another technique to assess myelin, and suggested that the latter might be more accurate and robust to quantify the myelin content in normal-appearing white matter [21].

Interestingly, T1 and T2 maps have been shown to highlight differences in the so-called normal-appearing parenchyma when comparing patients with multiple sclerosis and healthy controls. In particular, Vrenken *et al* demonstrated increased T1 values in normal-appearing white matter in all the patients with multiple sclerosis that were enrolled as part of their seminal study [22]. The increase in T1 was also shown in the normal-appearing grey matter, both cortical and deep (i.e. in the thalamus), supporting the theory that in patients with multiple sclerosis pathological changes can be found throughout the brain, also in regions that appear normal in conventional MRI. Manfredonia *et al* also demonstrated that T1 relaxometry is superior to conventional MRI in assessing disease progression and predicting prognosis in patients with primary progressive multiple sclerosis [23]. Indeed, although it was known that normal-appearing brain parenchyma had a role in the severity of the disability in patients with multiple sclerosis due to occult disease, as exemplified by the clinical MRI paradox, its previously difficult assessment became possible only thanks to the introduction of T1 mapping.

5.4.2 Proton spectroscopy

Proton MR spectroscopy (^{1}H-MRS) is a quantitative technique that can non-invasively measure brain metabolites *in vivo*. For a more comprehensive description of this technique and its application in multiple sclerosis see chapter 4, section 4.1. Briefly, several biological processes can be measured using ^{1}H-MRS, such as glucose consumption, variation in membrane turnover and proliferation [24, 25]. In patients with MS, the typical pattern of axonal damage is characterised by a decrease in *N*-acetylaspartate (NAA) and an increase in myo-inositol (mIns) concentrations [3].

5.4.3 Diffusion-weighted imaging

Diffusion-weighted imaging has had a central role in brain imaging since its inception. However, the assumption that diffusion within the brain parenchyma is isotropic is an over simplification and has been challenged by many authors over the past two decades. Indeed, the brain is a highly structured organ with axonal bundles dictating the potential directions for the diffusion of water molecules, resulting in different diffusion coefficients along different directions, so-called anisotropic diffusion. The latter is described by the diffusion tensor, a 3 × 3 matrix:

$$D = \begin{bmatrix} D_{xx} & D_{xy} & D_{xz} \\ D_{yx} & D_{yy} & D_{yz} \\ D_{zx} & D_{zy} & D_{zz} \end{bmatrix}.$$

In this matrix, D_{xx}, D_{yy} and D_{zz} represent the diffusion along the reference axis (x, y and z), while the six off-diagonal elements represent the correlation of random motions between each pair of principal directions. Diffusion tensor imaging (DTI) is a diffusion technique that probes this directionality [26]. Thanks to its quantitative nature, DTI can play a significant role in multiple sclerosis imaging. Decreased fractional anisotropy (a scalar expressing the degree of anisotropy) and increased mean diffusivity (a scalar of the diffusion in a given voxel) have been observed in demyelinating lesions as well as in areas of normal-appearing brain parenchyma as defined by conventional ^{1}H MRI [27, 28].

5.4.4 Magnetisation transfer

Magnetisation transfer (MT) is quantitative MRI technique based on the exchange of magnetisation between the free pool of protons and the pool bound to macromolecules, such as myelin or axonal membranes. Therefore, demyelination or axonal damage will result in alteration of the exchange between the two pools that is detectable with MT. The magnetisation transfer ratio (MTR) is a type of MT imaging in which two different sets of images are acquired, one without (MT_{off}) and one with (MT_{on}) the MT pulse. A ratio is then obtained by measuring the percentage difference between the two acquisitions [1]. MTR has been proved to be a reliable tool to detect demyelination and axonal loss [29–31], however, higher field strengths provide a higher SNR that results in a better spatial resolution and, therefore, better delineation of cortical demyelination. This improvement is more pronounced at ultra-high field strengths that allow the visualisation of subpial lesions [32].

5.4.5 Functional MRI

Since its inception, functional magnetic resonance imaging (fMRI) has been evaluated as a potential tool to assess functional changes in the motor and cognitive domains in patients with multiple sclerosis [33–36]. However, a great improvement resulted from the adoption of high- and ultra-high field magnets [37].

Chapter 3, section 3.1, is dedicated to fMRI, but briefly, this technique can play a role in assessing the direct damage to white and grey matter, but could also allow one to assess the adaptive brain functional reorganisation consequent to parenchymal damage, in particular if scans are obtained longitudinally during follow-up [38]. Furthermore, fMRI studies have suggested that functional cortical changes seen in patients with early relapsing-remitting MS can have an adaptive role in limiting the clinical impact of tissue injury [34]. A potential avenue for functional MRI in multiple sclerosis could be monitoring the effect of disease-modifying drugs. So far, few studies have delved into the potential application of this technique to monitor treatment, opening up a new niche for research and for establishing a novel biomarker.

5.4.6 Volumetric techniques

Multiple sclerosis is characterised by a brain volume decrease related to the loss of axons, neurons, glial cells and myelin. This is a progressive process, particularly in the absence of disease-modifying drugs, therefore interval changes in brain volume can be used to monitor the progression of multiple sclerosis and assess treatment response [39]. Volumetric analysis has been facilitated by the introduction of high field magnets (and ultra-high field more recently), thanks to the higher spatial resolution achievable by using higher fields (figure 5.2).

Brain volume has been assessed in its entirety, but also separately, looking at the white matter (WM) and grey matter (GM) components. Overall, brain volume is easier and quicker to measure without having to perform a segmentation to extrapolate white matter and grey matter. As it stands, brain atrophy has been

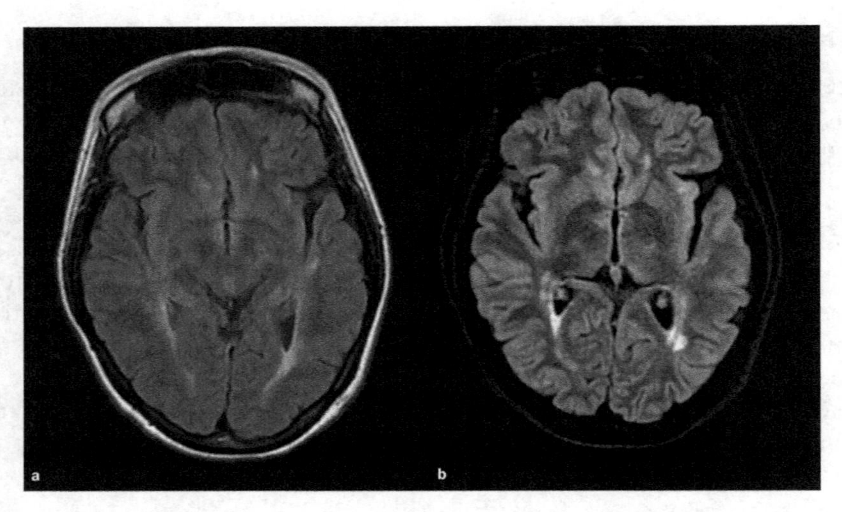

Figure 5.2. (a) 2D and (b) 3D FLAIR in a patient with multiple sclerosis. The 3D acquisition allows for better segmentation and quantification of the lesion burden thanks to the higher spatial resolution and the contiguity of the slices. Moreover, there is better separation between the contrast of grey and white matter, enhancing the differences between the two and allowing for an increase in the conspicuity of lesions for detection.

proven to accurately predict long term cognitive decline and disability in patients with multiple sclerosis with several studies reporting follow-up at 10 [40] and even 13 years [41]. Algorithm-based segmentation techniques allow for a probability-based separation between voxels which are likely to contain white matter and voxels which are likely to contain grey matter. There are several semi- and completely automated tools to perform segmentation and a description of these is outside the scope of this chapter, however, segmentation has uncovered the different behaviour of white matter and grey matter in multiple sclerosis and also the regional distribution of volume changes, for example associating memory impairment with mesial temporal volume loss. Moreover, grey matter volume loss is a stronger predictor of clinical disability, thus it has been proposed as a more accurate biomarker than overall brain atrophy.

5.5 New frontiers and future developments

Beyond proton imaging and spectroscopy, the increased SNR granted by moving from 1.5 T to 3.0 T makes the acquisition of lower natural abundance nuclei, such as phosphorus-31 (^{31}P), sodium-23 (^{23}Na) or carbon-13 (^{13}C), possible in clinically feasible scan times. As compared to ^{1}H, these nuclei prove less morphological and structural information, but allow the characterisation of metabolic processes within the cells. This characteristic is particularly welcome in multiple sclerosis imaging due to the lack of reliable strategies to assess early metabolic changes that could represent initial and potentially reversible alternations.

5.5.1 Phosphorus spectroscopy

Phosphorus (^{31}P) spectroscopy is a technique to probe inorganic and organic molecules with a phosphorus nucleus, such as adenosine triphosphate (ATP) and phosphocreatine (PCr). Using spectroscopic techniques, it is possible to probe the metabolism of organs, for example the heart, the liver, or the brain, in healthly subjects and in pathological conditions [42, 43]. Indeed, using a magnetisation transfer prepared phosphorus spectroscopy sequence, it is possible to measure metabolic flux through creatine kinase and ATP synthase [44]. Furthermore, with a pH-dependent chemical shift between inorganic phosphate and phosphocreatine, it is possible to provide a measure of intracellular pH (known to change in oncological and neurological disease) through ^{31}P spectroscopy [45].

However, there are a number of challenges to performing phosphorus spectroscopy at 1.5 T, which are somewhat elevated by moving to 3 T, mainly through the increased SNR. Due to the low natural concentration of organic molecules in the body, in the mmol L^{-1} range, such as ATP, there is a low natural signal available for NMR detection. This, in turn, leads to low SNR and long scan times at 1.5 T, prohibiting the use of ^{31}P in research or clinical examinations. However, moving to 3 T gives an increase in polarisation, as described in equation (5.1), and many studies have demonstrated the feasibility of acquiring ^{31}P data at higher field [46–48]. Nevertheless, even with this increase in SNR due to high field strength, large voxel sizes (commonly 10–30 mm^3) are used in acquisition, limiting the spatial sensitivity of the technique.

However, challenges are faced in the move from 1.5 T to 3 T in phosphorus acquisitions, with increased T1 for most metabolites, leading to longer repetition times between each excitation. This, in turn, leads to long scan times and the potential for introducing motion related artefacts in to spectra, in particular for unwell patients.

5.5.2 Sodium imaging

Sodium-23 is a quadrupolar nucleus that yields the second strongest nuclear magnetic resonance signal from biological tissues, after protons [49], however, MRI sensitivity is as low as 9.2% of proton sensitivity, resulting in an average SNR up to 20 000 times lower than the SNR for protons. With the wide availability of high field scanners, improvement in the design of radiofrequency coils and novel optimized sequences, ^{23}Na-MRI is now feasible with a temporal and spatial resolution that is clinically useful (figures 5.3 and 5.4) [50].

Several ^{23}Na-MRI studies have already been performed in the brain to evaluate the possible use of this technique for assessing tumours or neurodegenerative diseases both in a qualitative and quantitative fashion [51–60].

The first study assessing sodium MRI in patients with multiple sclerosis was published in 2010 by Inglese *et al* [54]. In her study, Inglese demonstrated that whilst the tissue sodium concentration in healthy controls was quite homogeneous, in patients with multiple sclerosis the concentration was increased both in enhancing and non-enhancing lesions, albeit the increase was more marked in the former. Since

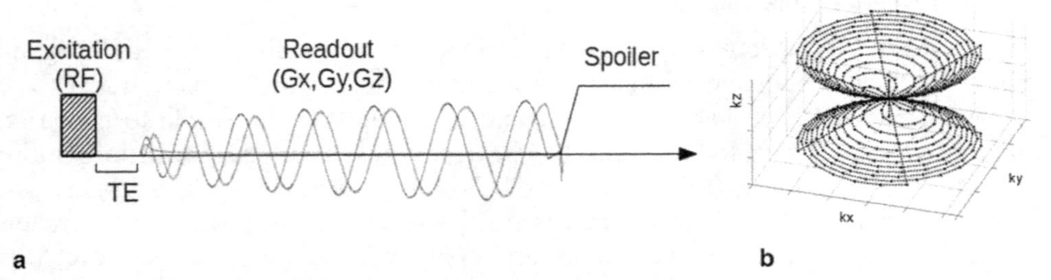

Figure 5.3. (a) Illustration of the MR pulse sequence used for sodium imaging at our institution. A state of the art sinusoidal read-out that encodes the image pixels is run at maximum slew rate to acquire the frequency spectrum at high speed using three perpendicular electromagnetic field gradients. The resulting data can be represented as sampled on cones (b) that will be run with different inclinations and offsets to fill a sphere which represents a full dataset.

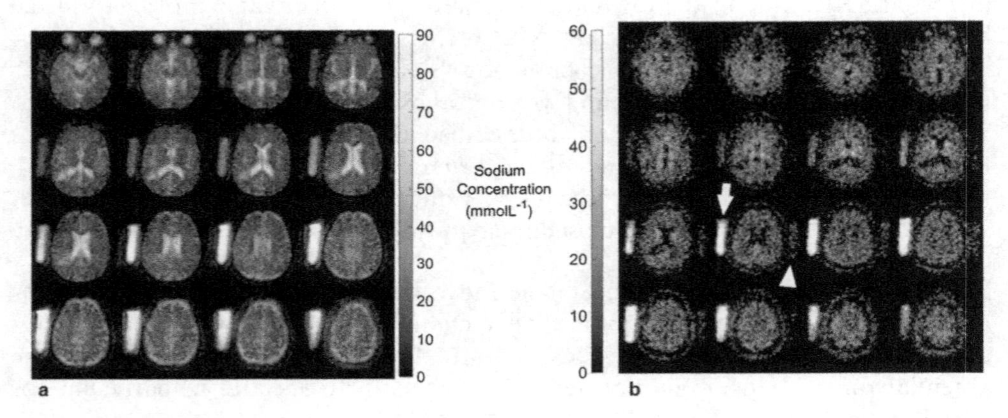

Figure 5.4. Example images of total sodium and intracellular weighted sodium in the MS brain. (a) Total sodium concentration map. (b) Iintracellular weighted sodium concentration map. Note the two phantoms with known sodium concentration next to the volunteer's head (more evident in (b); the arrow indicates the higher concentration phantom, the arrow head the lower concentration phantom) used to obtain the maps from the native acquisition. Adapted from [62].

then, more research groups have been focusing on this quantitative tool confirming the imbalance in sodium concentration in demyelinating lesions, but also in normal-appearing brain parenchyma in patients with secondary-progressive multiple sclerosis [61].

Our group developed a 3 mm isotropic sequence that was able to quantify the total sodium concentration in the entire brain with a scan time of about 12 min. Thanks to the high spatial resolution, we recently demonstrated for the first time intralesional sodium heterogeneity both in the intracellular and in the total sodium concentration (figure 5.5) [62]. The capability of assessing sodium concentration in the brain parenchyma in a non-invasive fashion will allow probing the biology of multiple sclerosis in unexplored ways, fostering our knowledge of the disease and improving how we monitor the status of the disease.

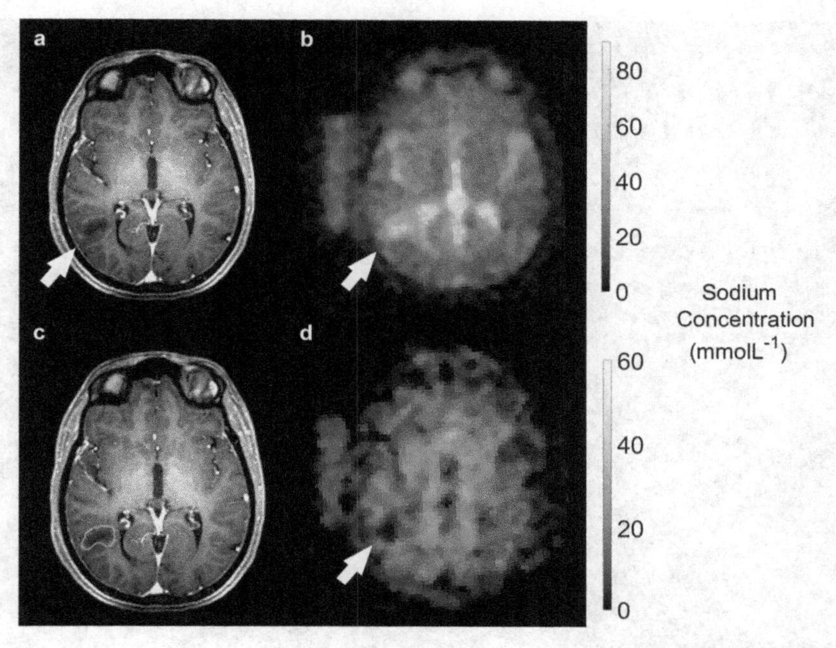

Figure 5.5. Proton and sodium images of the MS lesion and quantitative sodium analysis of the MS brain. (a) Post contrast-enhanced T1 weighted image; (b) total sodium map; (c) contour highlight of the progressing lesion; and (d) intracellular weighted (fluid suppressed) sodium map. The arrow denotes the active multiple sclerosis lesion on the post Gd T1 weighted image and sodium concentration maps. Adapted from [62].

5.5.3 Hyperpolarised ^{13}C MRSI

Since the chemical shift dispersion is magnetic field dependent, an increase in field strength results in an increased chemical shift dispersion, thus, the acquisition of novel techniques, such as hyperpolarised carbon-13 imaging, is currently being undertaken to assess the metabolism of both the healthy and oncological brain [63]. The capability of detecting signal from ^{13}C is also due to the improved sensitivity obtainable by transferring polarisation from an electron or nuclear spin that has a higher polarisation to the ^{13}C itself; a technique termed hyperpolarisation [64]. The currently most used technique for hyperpolarisation is the dynamic nuclear polarisation (DNP) and can increase the sensitivity by more than 10 000 times [65, 66]. DNP relies upon cooling down to 1 K a sample of a ^{13}C labelled compound before pulsing microwaves through it; after 2–3 h of hyperpolarisation, the sample is heated to body temperature before being injected into a subject [67].

Although there are many potential candidate molecules that can be labelled with ^{13}C and hyperpolarised with the DNP, the most promising molecule for brain imaging so far has been [1-^{13}C]pyruvate [68]. Results have so far been promising for estimating both the glycolytic flux of pyruvate to lactate as well as tricarboxylic acid metabolism signalled by the formation of bicarbonate both in pre-clinical models, healthy volunteers (figure 5.6) and in patients. An increased glycolytic flux paired with high cellular lactate excretion has been proven to distinguish a tumour from

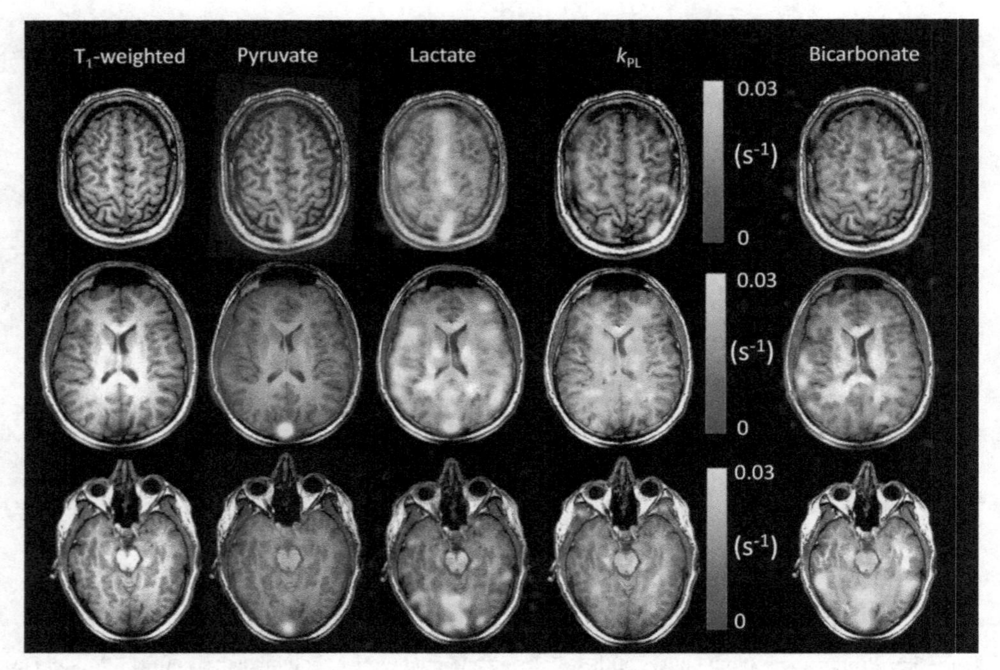

Figure 5.6. IDEAL spiral ^{13}C imaging demonstrating the metabolite distribution in the healthy human brain. Example summed images from the brain of a healthy volunteer demonstrating ^{13}C-pyruvate, ^{13}C-lactate and ^{13}C-bicarbonate signal from three axial slices: superior, central and inferior. The T1 weighted images have also been shown, as have the quantitative maps of the exchange of pyruvate to lactate (k_p in s^{-1}). Adapted from [78].

normal tissue, potentially improving tumour grade identification [68–70]. Translation from the bench to bedside was achieved at the University of California in San Francisco a few years ago with a seminal study in patients with prostate cancer [71]. Since then a few papers have been published demonstrating the *in vivo* detection of pyruvate and its metabolic cascade in humans, including primary and secondary brain tumours [72].

5.5.4 Magnetic resonance fingerprinting and synthetic magnetic resonance imaging

Magnetic resonance fingerprinting is a novel quantitative technique based on pseudorandomised acquisition that exploits the unique signal evolution or 'fingerprint' derived from the multiple material properties of the tissue under investigation [73]. After the acquisition, the post-processing after acquisition involves the use of dedicated pattern recognition algorithms to match the obtained fingerprints to a dictionary of predicted signal evolutions to translate the signal intensities into quantitative maps. This approach provides a robust, fully quantitative and multiparametric acquisition that can open up a new way of assessing tissues according to their specific characteristics [74]. Despite the great interest in this novel technique, so far there is only scant literature on neuroradiological applications. The first report on the use of magnetic resonance fingerprinting in patients with multiple sclerosis was featured in *Neurology* in 2016 [75]. In their preliminary study, Nakamura *et al* demonstrated that quantitative measurements obtained with magnetic resonance fingerprinting are able to differentiate patients with multiple sclerosis from healthy controls, distinguish disease courses and correlate with disability.

Synthetic magnetic resonance imaging aims to shorten the length of scan time without sacrificing the amount of information acquired [76]. This approach provides more information in the span of a single sequence, being able to create T1, T2 and proton density images from a single quantitative sequence. As an example of interest, Park *et al* demonstrated that the amount of myelin quantified using synthetic magnetic resonance imaging derived biomarkers was lower in cognitively impaired patients with and without white matter intensities on conventional T2 weighted images [77]. Moreover, the myelin content was independently associated with cognitive deficits. This study proposed the use of myelin quantification as a potential quantitative biomarker for cognitive dysfunction. Thus, synthetic magnetic resonance imaging can have a significant role in patients with multiple sclerosis, combining quicker scan times with added information compared to conventional imaging.

References

[1] Fox R J 2011 Advanced MRI in MS: current status and future challenges *Neurol. Clin.* **29** 357–80

[2] Kim J H *et al* 2006 Comparison of 1.5T and 3T1H MR spectroscopy for human brain tumors *Korean J. Radiol.* **7** 156–61

[3] Wattjes M P and Barkhof F 2009 High field MRI in the diagnosis of multiple sclerosis: high field-high yield? *Neuroradiology* **51** 279–92

[4] Keiper M D *et al* 1998 MR identification of white matter abnormalities in multiple sclerosis: a comparison between 1.5 T and 4 T *AJNR. Am. J. Neuroradiol.* **19** 1489–93

[5] Swanton J K *et al* 2007 MRI criteria for multiple sclerosis in patients presenting with clinically isolated syndromes: a multicentre retrospective study *Lancet Neurol.* **6** 677–86

[6] Wattjes M P *et al* 2008 Does high field MRI allow an earlier diagnosis of multiple sclerosis? *J. Neurol.* **255** 1159–63

[7] Wattjes M P *et al* 2006 Does high-field MR imaging have an influence on the classification of patients with clinically isolated syndromes according to current diagnostic MR imaging criteria for multiple sclerosis? *Am. J. Neuroradiol.* **27** 1794–8

[8] Lutterbey G *et al* 2007 Clinical evaluation of a speed optimized T2 weighted fast spin echo sequence at 3.0 T using variable flip angle refocusing, half-Fourier acquisition and parallel imaging *Br. J. Radiol.* **80** 668–73

[9] Umino M *et al* 2018 3D double inversion recovery MR imaging: clinical applications and usefulness in a wide spectrum of central nervous system diseases *J. Neuroradiol.* **46** 107–16

[10] Redpath T W and Smith F W 1994 Use of a double inversion recovery pulse sequence to image selectively grey or white brain matter *Br. J. Radiol.* **67** 1258–63

[11] Simon B *et al* 2010 Improved *in vivo* detection of cortical lesions in multiple sclerosis using double inversion recovery MR imaging at 3 tesla *Eur. Radiol.* **20** 1675–83

[12] Kollia K *et al* 2009 First clinical study on ultra-high-field MR imaging in patients with multiple sclerosis: Comparison of 1.5 T and 7 T *Am. J. Neuroradiol.* **30** 699–702
[13] Mainero C *et al* 2009 *In vivo* imaging of cortical pathology in multiple sclerosis using ultra-high field MRI *Neurology* **73** 941–8
[14] Madelin G, Oesingmann N and Inglese M 2010 Double inversion recovery MRI with fat suppression at 7 tesla: Initial experience *J. Neuroimaging* **20** 87–92
[15] Tintore M, Vidal-Jordana A and Sastre-Garriga J 2019 Treatment of multiple sclerosis—success from bench to bedside *Nat. Rev. Neurol.* **15** 53–8
[16] Petiet A, Adanyeguh I, Aigrot M S, Poirion E, Nait-Oumesmar B, Santin M and Stankoff B 2018 Ultra high field imaging of myelin disease models: towards specific markers of myelin integrity? *J. Comp. Neurol.* 1–11
[17] Koenig S H 1991 Cholesterol of myelin is the determinant of gray-white contrast in MRI of brain *Magn. Reson. Med.* **20** 285–91
[18] Deoni S C L 2011 Quantitative relaxometry of the brain *Top Magn. Reson. Imaging* **21** 101–13
[19] Stankiewicz J *et al* 2009 T1- and T2-based MRI measures of diffuse gray matter and white matter damage in patients with multiple sclerosis *J. Neuroimaging* **17** 16S–21S
[20] Laule C *et al* 2004 Water content and myelin water fraction in multiple sclerosis *J. Neurol.* **251** 284–93
[21] Tozer D J *et al* 2005 Correlation of apparent myelin measures obtained in multiple sclerosis patients and controls from magnetization transfer and multicompartmental T2 analysis *Magn. Reson. Med.* **53** 1415–22
[22] Vrenken H *et al* 2006 Whole-brain T1 mapping in multiple sclerosis: global changes of normal-appearing gray and white matter *Radiology* **240** 1–10
[23] Manfredonia F *et al* 2007 Normal-appearing brain T1 relaxation time predicts disability in early primary progressive multiple sclerosis *Arch. Neurol.* **64** 411–5
[24] Zhang H *et al* 2014 Role of magnetic resonance spectroscopy for the differentiation of recurrent glioma from radiation necrosis: a systematic review and meta-analysis *Eur. J. Radiol.* **83** 2181–9
[25] Price S J and Gillard J H 2011 Imaging biomarkers of brain tumour margin and tumour invasion *Br. J. Radiol.* **84** S159–67
[26] Hagmann P *et al* 2006 Central nervous system: state of the art understanding diffusion MR imaging techniques: from scalar diffusion-weighted imaging to diffusion tensor imaging and beyond *RadioGraphics* **26** 205–24
[27] Pagani E *et al* 2007 Diffusion MR imaging in multiple sclerosis: technical aspects and challenges *Am. J. Neuroradiol.* **28** 411–20
[28] Bester M *et al* 2008 Early anisotropy changes in the corpus callosum of patients with optic neuritis *Neuroradiology* **50** 549–57
[29] Schmierer K *et al* 2004 Magnetization transfer ratio and myelin in postmortem multiple sclerosis brain *Ann. Neurol.* **56** 407–15
[30] Fisniku L K *et al* 2011 UKPMC funders group magnetization transfer ratio abnormalities reflect clinically relevant grey matter damage in multiple sclerosis *Mult. Scler.* **15** 668–77
[31] Samson R S *et al* 2014 Investigation of outer cortical magnetisation transfer ratio abnormalities in multiple sclerosis clinical subgroups *Mult. Scler.* **20** 1322–30

[32] Abdel-Fahim R *et al* 2014 Improved detection of focal cortical lesions using 7 T magnetisation transfer imaging in patients with multiple sclerosis *Mult. Scler. Relat. Disord.* **3** 258–65

[33] Yousry T A, Berry I and Filippi M 1998 Functional magnetic resonance imaging in multiple sclerosis *J. Neurol. Neurosurg. Psychiatry* **64** S85–7

[34] Audoin B *et al* 2003 Compensatory cortical activation observed by fMRI during a cognitive task at the earliest stage of multiple sclerosis *Hum. Brain Mapp.* **20** 51–8

[35] Parry A M M *et al* 2003 Potentially adaptive functional changes in cognitive processing for patients with multiple sclerosis and their acute modulation by rivastigmine *Brain* **126** 2750–60

[36] Mainero C *et al* 2004 Enhanced brain motor activity in patients with MS after a single dose of 3,4-diaminopyridine *Neurology* **62** 2044–50

[37] Uğurbil K *et al* 2013 Pushing spatial and temporal resolution for functional and diffusion MRI in the Human Connectome Project *Neuroimage* **80** 80–104

[38] Enzinger C *et al* 2015 Longitudinal fMRI studies: exploring brain plasticity and repair in MS *Mult. Scler.* **22** 269–78

[39] Sinnecker T *et al* 2018 Future brain and spinal cord volumetric imaging in the clinic for monitoring treatment response in MS *Curr. Treat. Options Neurol.* **20** 17

[40] Jacobsen C *et al* 2014 Brain atrophy and disability progression in multiple sclerosis patients: a 10-year follow-up study *J. Neurol. Neurosurg. Psychiatry* **85** 1109–15

[41] Filippi M *et al* 2013 Gray matter damage predicts the accumulation of disability 13 years later in MS *Neurology* **81** 1759–67

[42] Lin G and Chung Y L 2014 Current opportunities and challenges of magnetic resonance spectroscopy, positron emission tomography, and mass spectrometry imaging for mapping cancer metabolism *in vivo Biomed Res. Int.* **2014** 625095

[43] Harper D G, Jensen J E and Renshaw P F 2016 Phosphorus spectroscopy (31P MRS) of the brain in psychiatric disorders *eMagRes* **5** 1257–70

[44] Liu Y, Gu Y and Yu X 2017 Assessing tissue metabolism by phosphorous-31 magnetic resonance spectroscopy and imaging: a methodology review *Quant. Imaging Med. Surg.* **7** 707–16

[45] Cichocka M, Kozub J and Urbanik A 2015 PH measurements of the brain using phosphorus magnetic resonance spectroscopy (31PMRS) in healthy men—comparison of two analysis methods polish *J. Radiol.* **80** 509–14

[46] Novak J *et al* 2014 Clinical protocols for ^{31}P MRS of the brain and their use in evaluating optic pathway gliomas in children *Eur. J. Radiol.* **83** e106–12

[47] Panda A *et al* 2012 Phosphorus liver MRSI at 3 T using a novel dual-tuned eight-channel ^{31}P/^{1}H coil *Magn. Reson. Med.* **68** 1346–56

[48] Hakkarainen A *et al* 2017 Metabolic profile of liver damage in non-cirrhotic virus C and autoimmune hepatitis: a proton decoupled ^{31}P-MRS study *Eur. J. Radiol.* **90** 205–11

[49] Madelin G and Regatte R R 2013 Biomedical applications of sodium MRI *in vivo J. Magn. Reson. Imaging* **38** 511–29

[50] Konstandin S and Nagel A M 2014 Measurement techniques for magnetic resonance imaging of fast relaxing nuclei *Magn. Reson. Mater. Phys. Biol. Med.* **27** 5–19

[51] Inglese M *et al* 2013 Sodium imaging as a marker of tissue injury in patients with multiple sclerosis *Mult. Scler. Relat. Disord.* **2** 263–9

[52] Zaaraoui W *et al* 2012 Distribution of brain sodium accumulation correlates with disability in multiple sclerosis: a cross-sectional ^{23}Na MR imaging study *Radiology* **264** 859–67
[53] Yushmanov V E *et al* 2013 Correlated sodium and potassium imbalances within the ischemic core in experimental stroke: a ^{23}Na MRI and histochemical imaging study *Brain Res.* **1527** 199–208
[54] Inglese M *et al* 2010 Brain tissue sodium concentration in multiple sclerosis: a sodium imaging study at 3 tesla *Brain* **133** 847–57
[55] Reetz K *et al* 2012 Increased brain tissue sodium concentration in Huntington's Disease—a sodium imaging study at 4 T *Neuroimage* **63** 517–24
[56] Nagel A M *et al* 2011 The potential of relaxation-weighted sodium magnetic resonance imaging as demonstrated on brain tumors *Invest. Radiol.* **46** 539–47
[57] Mellon E A a *et al* 2009 Sodium MR imaging detection of mild Alzheimer disease: preliminary study *AJNR Am. J. Neuroradiol.* **30** 978–84
[58] Thulborn K R *et al* 2009 Quantitative sodium MR imaging and sodium bioscales for the management of brain tumors *Neuroimaging Clin. N. Am.* **19** 615–24
[59] Haneder S *et al* 2015 ^{23}Na-MRI of recurrent glioblastoma multiforme after intraoperative radiotherapy: technical note *Neuroradiology* **57** 321–6
[60] Ouwerkerk R, Bleich K and Gillen J 2003 Tissue sodium concentration in human brain tumors as measured with ^{23}Na MR imaging *Radiology* **23** 529–37
[61] Paling D *et al* 2013 Sodium accumulation is associated with disability and a progressive course in multiple sclerosis *Brain* **136** 2305–17
[62] Grist J T *et al* 2018 Imaging intralesional heterogeneity of sodium concentration in multiple sclerosis: Initial evidence from ^{23}Na-MRI *J. Neurol. Sci.* **387** 111–4
[63] Zaccagna F *et al* 2018 Hyperpolarized carbon-13 magnetic resonance spectroscopic imaging: a clinical tool for studying tumour metabolism *Br. J. Radiol.* **2017** 20170688
[64] Månsson S *et al* 2006 ^{13}C imaging—a new diagnostic platform *Eur. Radiol.* **16** 57–67
[65] Ardenkjaer-Larsen J H *et al* 2003 Increase in signal-to-noise ratio of > 10 000 times in liquid-state NMR *Proc. Natl. Acad. Sci. USA* **100** 10158–63
[66] Brindle K M *et al* 2011 Tumor imaging using hyperpolarized ^{13}C magnetic resonance spectroscopy *Magn. Reson. Med.* **66** 505–19
[67] Brindle K M 2015 Imaging metabolism with hyperpolarized ^{13}C-labeled cell substrates *J. Am. Chem. Soc.* **137** 6418–27
[68] Albers M J *et al* 2008 Hyperpolarized ^{13}C lactate, pyruvate, and alanine: noninvasive biomarkers for prostate cancer detection and grading *Cancer Res.* **68** 8607–15
[69] Golman K *et al* 2006 Metabolic imaging by hyperpolarized ^{13}C magnetic resonance imaging for *in vivo* tumor diagnosis *Cancer Res.* **66** 10855–60
[70] Park I *et al* 2010 Hyperpolarized ^{13}C magnetic resonance metabolic imaging: application to brain tumors *Neuro. Oncol.* **12** 133–44
[71] Nelson S J *et al* 2013 Metabolic imaging of patients with prostate cancer using hyper-polarized [$^{1\text{-}13}$C]pyruvate *Sci. Transl. Med.* **5** 198ra108
[72] Miloushev V Z *et al* 2018 Metabolic imaging of the human brain with hyperpolarized ^{13}C Pyruvate demonstrates ^{13}C lactate production in brain tumor patients *Cancer Res.* **78** 3755–60
[73] Ma D *et al* 2013 Magnetic resonance fingerprinting *Nature* **495** 187–93
[74] European Society of Radiology 2015 Magnetic resonance fingerprinting—a promising new approach to obtain standardized imaging biomarkers from MRI *Insights Imaging* **6** 163–5

[75] Nakamura K *et al* 2016 A novel method for quantification of normal appearing brain tissue in multiple sclerosis: magnetic resonance fingerprinting *Neurology* **86** P4.158
[76] Smedby O *et al* 2012 Synthetic MRI of the brain in a clinical setting *Acta Radiol.* **53** 1158–63
[77] Park M, Moon Y, Han S H, Kim H K and Moon W J 2018 Myelin loss in white matter hyperintensities and normal-appearing white matter of cognitively impaired patients: a quantitative synthetic magnetic resonance imaging study *Eur. Radiol.* doi: 10.1007/s00330-018-5836-x
[78] Grist J T *et al* 2019 Quantifying normal human brain metabolism using hyperpolarized [$^{1\text{-}13}$C]pyruvate and magnetic resonance imaging *Neuroimage* **189** 171–9

IOP Publishing

Neurological Disorders and Imaging Physics, Volume 1
Application of multiple sclerosis
Luca Saba and Jasjit S Suri

Chapter 6

Applications of nuclear medicine in multiple sclerosis

Giuseppe Corrias, Jasjit S Suri and Luca Saba

When applied to the brain, nuclear medicine (NM) techniques may reveal critical information about the most devastating diseases, from multiple sclerosis (MS) to Alzheimer's to traumatic brain injury.

NM is an imaging modality which utilizes radiopharmaceuticals to generate an image. Most of the radiopharmaceuticals are composed of a radioactive isotope (which emits the radioactivity used to create images) bound to a biologically active ligand. Radiopharmaceuticals are typically injected intravenously. NM has the advantage of being able to explore physiological processes that are naturally happening within the organism, such as blood flow, glucose uptake and binding of neurotransmitters. However, the obtained images have a lower spatial resolution than other imaging modalities, thus integration with computed tomography (CT) or magnetic resonance (MR) is required.

6.1 Physical and physiological considerations for a nuclear medicine study

6.1.1 Gamma camera

Traditional nuclear medicine uses a crystal detector NaI(Tl) which scintillates (gives out a short burst of light) on exposure to radiation. Photomultiplier tubes or photodiodes positioned adjacent to the crystal will amplify and convert the weak light signal emitted by the scintillator crystal to electrons. These electrons are then fed into a computer to generate an image. The collimator is a device to channel the radiation (gamma rays or photons) produced by the radiopharmaceuticals in an appropriate direction to the crystal detector.

doi:10.1088/2053-2563/ab1fdcch6

6.1.2 Photon energy

The optimum energy for detection of photons is around 150 keV using the conventional gamma camera. In practice, the useful energy is between 50 keV and 300 keV. Below this energy, much of the emitted radiation is absorbed within the patient. Photons which are too high in energy will penetrate a standard scintillator crystal without producing a useful image. A thicker and denser crystal will be needed.

6.1.3 Half-life

The radioactive half-life can be defined as the time in which radiation emission decreases by a half and is an important feature in NM. It governs the ideal time to image and the dose of radiopharmaceuticals given to the patients. By understanding the half-life of a radiopharmaceutical, one can utilize its properties to study various physiological processes. Materials with a very short half-life can be imaged instantaneously but require a high initial dose to be given to patients. The disadvantage of such reagents with a short half-life is that their production must occur close to the patient. This makes them costly and inconvenient to use. Materials with a very long half-life are useful in imaging over a period of time. However, patients remain radioactive for a considerable time and the initial dose of radiopharmaceutical has to be kept low, which could compromise the quality of the images.

6.1.4 Production of radiopharmaceuticals

The isotope most commonly used in conventional NM is technetium-99m (99mTc) because it emits gamma radiation of an easily detectable energy (140 keV) and has a biologically useful half-life (6 h). It is produced from a molybdenum-99/technetium-99m generator. The generator is portable; it can be purchased and stored in a secured unit in the hospital. Production of PET isotopes requires an expensive, large machine called a cyclotron which accelerates subatomic particles to nearly the speed of light. The particles or protons then collide against a target to produce an unstable positron emitter isotope.

6.1.5 Imaging

Using the planar view is a useful method to give an overview of large parts of the body, e.g. bone, lung and renal scintigrams, but brain imaging requires more precise definitions. Therefore, the planar view is rarely used in routine brain studies. Single photon emission tomography, (SPET; also known as single photon emission computed tomography, SPECT) is a method using data from gamma radiation obtained over 360° for multiplanar reconstructions similar to MR images. Positron emission tomography (PET) is a technique which uses isotopes which undergo an annihilation reaction. Certain nuclei of the radioactive material emit positrons (anti-electrons). On collision with electrons, both the positron and electron are annihilated and two gamma rays are emitted, each with an energy of 511 keV. Conveniently for imaging, the gamma rays are emitted at exactly 180°, which allows back projection for precise localization of the source of emission.

6.1.6 Nuclear medicine imaging tracers for neurology

Tracers to investigate neurological disorders using PET or SPECT have found many applications (see table 6.1). Several molecular targets can be studied *in vivo* in humans in combination with pathophysiological conditions. Most attention has been given to tracers for the investigation of the role of translocator protein (TSPO), the deposition of beta-amyloid and the dopaminergic system. For these targets, many clinical studies have been published with the application of a variety of tracers. Other targets of interest that have been studied in man to a lesser extent are receptors for *N*-methyl-D-aspartate acid (NMDA), the serotonergic system, receptors for adenosine, gamma-aminobutyric acid (GABA), opioids, metabotropic glutamate receptor subtype 5 (mGlu-5) and tracers for the cholinergic system. In addition, several transporter systems have received a great deal of attention. Many other tracers are under development for new molecular targets, opening new horizons in the future. An ideal nuclear medicine imaging tracer for brain imaging should fulfill the following criteria:

- A simple automated synthesis procedure suitable for reliable production and low radiation burden for personnel. For clinical studies, GMP compliance is a prerequisite.
- Appropriate specific activity which should be sufficiently high that binding of the tracers is minimally affected by nonradioactive counterparts. In particular for targets with low densities, high specific activity is an important issue.
- $\log P$ between 1.5 and 4 in order to passively penetrate the lipophilic blood–brain barrier enabling high accumulation of target bound radioactivity.
- High affinity (expressed as B_{max}/K_D) to achieve sufficient radioactive signal bound at the target and high specificity so that measured radioactive signal represents binding to the target of interest.
- Metabolic stability to ensure that measured radioactivity represents binding of the administered tracer and not the metabolite.

6.2 Clinical developments

6.2.1 Cerebrovascular disease

The assessment of early stroke has always been an important aim for NM. Almost immediately after the onset of the vascular insult, functional and metabolic abnormalities can be detected by NM modalities. It was through early studies with ^{15}O water PET that hypoperfusion was classified into three stages: irreversible cerebral infarction occurring with cerebral blood flow (CBF) < 7–12 ml/100 g min^{-1} (ischemic core), abnormally functioning but viable tissue with the potential for recovery or progression to infarction with CBF < 20 ml/100 g min^{-1} but above the infarction threshold (penumbra), and mildly hypoperfused but otherwise normally functioning

Table 6.1. Nuclear medicine imaging tracers for neurology.

Target	Related disease	Tracers (human application)	Binding mechanism
TSPO	MS, AD, stroke, PD, HD, schizophrenia	[^{11}C]PK11195, DAA and PBR derivatives	Antagonist
GABA	Stroke	[^{11}C]Flumazenil	Antagonist
Dopaminergic system	PD, HD, tardive dyskinesia, schizophrenia, autism, ADHD, drug abuse, depression	[^{18}F]FDOPA, [^{11}C]SCH23390 [^{11}C]Raclopride [^{11}C]PHNOù [^{11}C]-Beta-CIT, PE2I	Vesicular storage Dopamine transporter D1 antagonist D2 agonist and antagonist
β-amyloid	AD, MCI	[^{11}C]PIB	Staining agent
NMDA	Schizophrenia	[^{11}C]GSK-931145	Antagonist
P-glycoprotein	Neurodegeneration	[^{11}C]Verapamil, [^{11}C]dLop	Substrate
Cholinergic system	AD, PD, HD, schizophrenia	[^{11}C]MP4A [^{18}F]TZTP	Acetylcholinesterase inhibitor, M2 antagonist
mGlu-5	Depression, anxiety, schizophrenia, PD	[^{11}C]ABP688	Antagonist
VMAT	PD, AD, HD	[^{11}C]DTPZ	
Adenosine receptor	PD, AD, epilepsy, sleep, neuroinflammation	[^{11}C]MPDX [^{11}C]TSMX	A1 antagonist A2a antagonist
Serotonergic system	Depression, anxiety, OCD, schizophrenia	[^{11}C]DASB [^{11}C]WAY100635 [^{11}C]MDL100907	Serotonin transporter 5-HT 1A antagonist 5-HT 2A antagonist
Norephedrine	Depression	[^{11}C]Methylreboxetine	NE transporter
Opioid receptors	Analgesia, shock, appetite, thermoregulation	[^{11}C]Diprenorphine	Kappa receptor antagonist
Monoamine oxidase	Neurodegenerative and inflammatory processes	[^{11}C]Deprenyl [^{11}C]Harmine	MAO inhibitors
Energy	Neurodegenerative and inflammatory processes	[^{18}F]FDG	Glucose consumption
Neuronal activity	Neurodegenerative and inflammatory processes	[^{15}O]water	Blood flow

and not at-risk tissue with CBF > 20–22 (oligemia; normal CBF is 50–55 ml/100 g min^{-1}) [1, 2]. The proposed role of SPECT in acute stroke is in principle in patient selection for thrombolytic therapy, from which only few patients ultimately benefit, by identification of the potentially salvageable penumbra. The two commonly used radiotracers are 99mTc HMPAO (Ceretec), which is only the Food and Drug

Administration approved radiotracer for detecting altered rCBF in stroke, and 99mTc ECD (Neurolite), which is approved as an adjunct in acute stroke imaging after diagnosis is confirmed by other modalities. SPECT imaging confers early sensitivity in acute stroke—90% of patients seen within 8 h have perfusion abnormalities, which is higher than with plain CT, with sensitivities among SPECT, CT and magnetic resonance imaging (MRI) becoming similar at 72 h [3]. Treatment of acute stroke encompasses supportive measures as well as interventional strategies, with the overall goal of improving survival and quality of life. Interventions include intravenous thrombolytic therapy with a tissue-type plasminogen activator, endovascular therapies, including intra-arterial thrombolytic administration and clot retrieval procedures, and surgical decompression in patients with malignant stroke [4]. These treatments target the ischemic penumbra, whose perfusion lies between the thresholds of infarction and neuronal impairment, which is at risk of becoming included within the expanding ischemic core. Proper treatment of areas of misery perfusion within the penumbra prevents further deterioration of the clinical outcome, while salvaging the penumbra is the main determinant of neurologic recovery [5]. Although the treatment window is currently limited to 4.5 h because of a reduced chance of penumbral salvage and increased risk of hemorrhage, cerebral edema and death beyond this window [6], early studies with PET indicated that penumbra with misery perfusion may be viable, at least in some cases, for up to 48 h.

At present, stroke triage algorithms do not incorporate nuclear imaging into acute treatment decisions, primarily because of the technical challenge of performing such a 1 h study in a short time window. However, several studies have demonstrated the potential utility and, in light of the extended treatment window, potential feasibility of nuclear imaging in this setting—in particular if faster and/or dual scanning procedures are developed. The recent DAWN trial showed how outcomes can be improved in selected patients with a mismatch between clinical deficit and infarct when treated with Thrombectomy 6–24 h after stroke [7]. Baird *et al* [8] demonstrated that in patients undergoing reperfusion therapy in ischemic stroke, the percentage improvement in perfusion derangements on resting perfusion HMPAO SPECT from 24 to 48 h is strongly correlated with stroke scores at 3 months, corroborating the efforts toward treatment during the early reperfusion window.

In large part, the evaluation of the isochemic penumbra has been supplanted by the use of perfusion- and diffusion-weighted MRI (perfusion-weighted imaging PWI/DWI mismatch) in both clinical and research settings to both select patients for therapy and monitor response to treatment. However, although clinically useful for patient management, the PWI/DWI mismatch does not reliably delineate the penumbra as defined by ^{15}O PET measures, largely because of the sensitivity of the PWI sequence to acquisition parameters [9].

6.2.2 Neurodegenerative disorders

Recently, European guidelines for using PET-CT in diagnosing dementia have been issued to help clinicians to adapt the issues of evidence quality to FDG-PET diagnostic studies and assess the evidence available in the current literature to assist in making recommendations for clinical use [10]. The commonly used criteria for diagnosis are still based on clinical and exclusion criteria, and no single specific test is available [11].

PET imaging is highly specific for investigating molecular markers of neuro-inflammatory processes such as multiple sclerosis. The most extensively investigated molecular target is the 18 KDa translocator protein (TSPO). Autoradiography studies have suggested that TSPO density mainly reflects activated microglia in multiple sclerosis patients' brains. It has been proven how PET studies show a higher TSPO signal in the white and gray matter of MS patients, that correlates with disease severity. With the latest developments and the validation of a wider range of molecular targets, the impact of PET imaging on the progress of neurobiological research in MS has become crucial.

Translocator protein TSPO (formerly called the peripheral benzodiazepine receptor)

The microglia constitute about 10% of the total brain cell population and represent the main form of immune defense in the CNS [12]. Microglia become activated after an injury occurs within the CNS, and they can be identified and distinguished from their resting phenotype based on a combination of morphological and immunophenotypic changes [13]. This microglia activation correlates with neuroinflammation, which plays an important role in the onset of neurodegenerative disease. Microglial activation up-regulates the expression of the TSPO, formerly known as the peripheral benzodiazepine receptor (PBR) that is involved in the release of proinflammatory cytokines during inflammation and is present at very low levels in the normal healthy CNS [14]. The up-regulation of TSPO expression can be detected *in vivo* with PET and selective radioligands, several of which have been developed [14]. [^{11}C]PK11195 [1-(2-chlorophenyl)-*N*-methyl-*N*-(1-methylpropyl)-3-isoquinoline carboxamide] is the first non-benzodiazepine and selective TSPO PET ligand [15]. [^{11}C]PK11195 has affinity for TSPO up to the nanomolar concentration [16]. Increased brain uptake of [^{11}C]PK11195 has been used mainly for assessing microglia/macrophage activation as an indication of neuronal and tissue damage in various neurodegenerative disorders, including multiple sclerosis, Alzheimer's disease (AD), Parkinson's disease (PD), amyotrophic lateral sclerosis, Huntington's disease, HIV, herpes encephalitis and schizophrenia. Although this tracer shows increased brain uptake in several neurodegenerative disorders, such as MS, AD, PD, Huntington's disease, HIV, herpes encephalitis and schizophrenia, it lacks sensitivity and specificity. These problems have jeopardized the development of a standard quantitative method of analysis. For this reason, other TSPO tracers have been developed, and are under investigation. Many research efforts in preclinical studies are aimed at the following issues: (i) the metabolic stability of the tracer, (ii) the binding potential (BP), (iii) ligand receptor kinetics and (iv) quantitation methods. Most of these human studies used a reference tissue to measure the uptake of radioactivity.

Neuroimaging hallmarks of MS

Multiple sclerosis (MS) is a chronic debilitating disease and the most common cause of nontraumatic neurological disability in young adults. The most common presentation of the disease (about 80% of patients) involves an initial diagnosis of relapsing–remitting MS (RRMS), and patients experience relapses followed by periods of remission. Relapses usually last no more than a few months, and the patient regains neurological function. As the disease progresses, typically after 15–20 years around 65% of this group of patients enters the secondary progressive phase (SPMS), which is characterized by a steady progression of neurological symptoms [17]. The remaining 20% of individuals who develop MS present with abrupt progression from disease onset, known as primary progressive MS (PPMS). The signs and symptoms are variable, including sensory, motor, visual, cognitive and emotional changes. Pathologically, MS is characterized by the presence of neuroinflammation, demyelination and neurodegeneration at different sites within the central nervous system (CNS). Focal areas of demyelination in which myelin, oligodendrocytes and axons are destroyed by inflammation cause the reversible disability in RRMS. The blood–brain barrier is disrupted, and lesion areas become more edematous. The resolution of inflammation and demyelination contributes to the clinical recovery and remission.

Historically, MS has been considered as a white matter disorder, however, the latest histopathological investigations have shown the presence of gray matter pathology in the cortex and deep nuclei, which becomes more prominent as the disease advances [18, 19]. There is evidence that gray matter pathological changes that importantly contribute to clinical disease severity are already present in the early stages of the disease and become more prominent when the disease progresses. This is well shown by a study which used [^{11}C]PK11195 in patients with RRMS and SPMS, proving an increased cortical gray matter TSPO expression that correlates clinically with levels of neurological disability.

Currently, the most widely available imaging tool to diagnose MS is magnetic resonance imaging (MRI). MRI has an established role in highlighting *in vivo* biomarkers of MS and has been used as the gold standard to investigate the natural course of the disease and monitor treatment response in clinical studies [20]. In RRMS patients, the effects of treatment on lesions visible on MRI and their effects on the frequency of relapses are strongly correlated, supporting the use of MRI parameters as surrogates for clinical end points [20]. However, a reduction in lesion size on MRI of inflammatory activity correlates weakly with disability regression in SPMS. At high levels of disability, there are no connections between the number and size of T2 weighted hyperintensities and degree of disability, indicating that other factors should be considered when assessing the more advanced phase of the disease. Although data derived from autopsies suggest widespread cortical involvement in MS, it is not possible to assess the contribution of cortical pathology with MRI imaging techniques. T1 and T2 weighted MRI sequences detect only a minority of cortical lesions. This different appearance on MRI may be due to the different inflammatory cell infiltration of cortical gray matter lesions. Another reason could be an absence of blood–brain barrier damage in cortical gray matter lesions. The detection of periventricular and juxtacortical lesions has a very high sensitivity with double inversion recovery (DIR) and phase sensitive inversion recovery; however, intracortical lesions remain difficult to detect even with these recent MR techniques. With the use of high field 7 T, detection of cortical lesions improves greatly [21]. However, disclosing extensive subpial demyelination with MRI remains challenging. Another important drawback of MRI is the impossibility of differentiating hyperintense lesions on T2 weighted images, in particular between reflect edema, demyelination, or astrogliosis. For these reasons it is hard to transform the clinical diagnosis of MS and develop a deeper knowledge on the neuropathology of this disease with only the use of MRI.

On the other hand, nuclear medicine with PET offers a powerful noninvasive technique, which allows biochemical analysis of brain processes, and it also allows functional mapping of brain tissue activity. In research, PET has led to a deeper understanding of MS through *in vivo* investigations of underlying pathophysiology.

The high specificity of biological targets of PET radioligands has been used to find the basic mechanisms in MS pathophysiology, which can be grouped into: neuroinflammation and activated microglia; demyelination and remyelination; brain activation and metabolism; and the cannabinoid, gamma-aminobutyric acid (GABA) and adenosinergic systems in MS. The most extensively characterized target is the 18 KDa translocator protein (TSPO), which has been linked to neuroinflammation and activated microglia. Preliminary evidence also indicates the potential use of the adenosine 2A receptors (A2ARs) and some myelin components. Other targets hold promise for future applications, for example, receptors such as GABA A, cannabinoid CB 2, acetylcholine, and some purinergic receptors and cellular components such as phosphatidylserine.

The 18 kDA translocator protein (TSPO)

The peripheral benzodiazepine receptor (PBR) was first discovered as a different benzodiazepine receptor from the classic receptor found in the CNS. TSPO is primarily found on the outer mitochondrial membrane, but it is localized also in the cell membrane and in the nucleus and perinuclear area in different cell lines [22]. TSPO has different functions, the most important being cholesterol transport control from the cytoplasm to the mitochondria (where steroid synthesis takes place) in the steroid synthesis pathway. Other physiological functions attributed to TSPO are cell growth and proliferation, heme biosynthesis, control of apoptosis, synthesis of bile acids, calcium flow, mitochondrial respiration and embryonic development. However, one of the most important activities of TSPO related to nuclear medicine and MS is chemotaxis and cellular immunity and is strictly connected to neuroinflammation and activated microglia: during an inflammatory response the expression of TSPO is upregulated, causing the release of proinflammatory cytokines. This mechanism is present at very low levels in the normal healthy CNS. A number of endogenous ligands that bind to TSPO have been discovered: the diazepam binding inhibitor (DBI) or endozepine; cholesterol; and porphyrins (protoporphyrin IX, mesoporphyrin IX, deuteroporphyrin IX, hemin). In healthy subjects TSPO is expressed in steroid-synthetizing peripheral tissues. Research by

Cosenza-Nashat *et al* [23] mapped localization and the degree of expression of TSPO with immunohistochemistry in the postmortem brain tissue of healthy subjects. The main expression of TSPO was found within macrophages and microglia, astrocytes, oligodendrocytes, endothelial cells and smooth muscle cells. TSPO was also present in subpial and subependymal glia, meninges (vessels, macrophages and sometimes arachnoid cells), ependymal cells and choroid plexus. Some punctate staining was found in neuronal cell bodies as well.

Rationale for imaging of activated microglia in MS

Microglia, cells from the mesodermal cell line, constitute about 10% of the total brain cell population and represent the main form of resident immune defense in the CNS [24]. In the healthy CNS these cells have a ramified morphology, a small soma with fine cellular processes. Many potential brain insults may cause microglial activation: infection, trauma, ischemia, neurodegenerative diseases, or altered neuronal activity. All these insults can evoke rapid and profound changes in the microglial cell shape, gene expression and the functional behavior. In this way, hours to days after CNS injury, microglia become activated, and they can be identified and distinguished from their resting phenotype based on a combination of morphological, immunophenotypic and, most importantly for nuclear medicine, protein expression changes [13]. The synthesis of proteins, such as chemoattractive factors, secreted to the intercellular CNS space, recruits and guides immune cell populations, and stimulates the presentation of antigens to T cells which can subsequently aid in adaptive immunity. Microglia also have phagocytotic activities, useful to clear tissue debris, damaged cells, or antibody-coated and opsonized antigens. Finally, microglia synthesize and secrete potential neurotoxins that may cause neuronal damage [25]. The microglia inflammatory response can be divided into acute and chronic: the acute response is generally beneficial because it minimizes injury and promotes tissue repair by releasing neuroinflammatory mediators such as TNF, IL-1 and IL-6 [26, 27]. In contrast, chronic neuroinflammation with continuous microglial activation has detrimental consequences in chronic neuroinflammatory disorders such as MS.

It has been known for decades that in MS, the areas of tissue damage and demyelination are rich in activated microglia, giving nuclear medicine techniques a unique opportunity for imaging the pathological processes underlying MS, with ligands addressed by TSPO.

As seen above, microglia activation contributes to the inflammation underlying MS through several mechanisms, such as the presentation of antigens and the secretion of proinflammatory cytokines, initiating an acute inflammatory response. A peculiar characteristic of microglia in the pathophysiology of MS is the clearance of damaged tissue, a property potentially linked both to recovery of function and to RRMS. Microglia may also exert a protective function in MS as they can promote tissue regeneration and repair. A very important point, for which nuclear medicine has claimed its superiority against MRI, is that activated microglia may represent an early stage of tissue injury, which precedes the formation of demyelinated plaques. Finally, it has been proven that cortical lesions include significant activated microglia. Therefore, imaging activated microglia can characterize neuroinflammatory involvement in normal-appearing white matter and in cortical gray matter, with the possibility of both predicting disease progression and studying the relationship between cortical pathology and related clinical symptoms, such as emotional and cognitive changes.

PET studies using TSPO ligands in MS patients
The TSPO ligands, studied to date in PET studies involving patients with MS, are [^{11}C]PK11195, [^{11}C]vinpocetine, [^{11}C]PBR28 and [^{18}F]FEDAA1106. The most well-characterized radiotracer is [^{11}C]PK11195. The other radioligands alongside other second-generation TSPO radioligands, such as ^{11}C-DAA1106 and ^{18}F-FEDAA1106,32Y34, were developed to address limitations associated with the application of ^{11}C-PK11195 PET, including a high level of nonspecific binding [28] and a poor signal-to-noise ratio, which complicates quantification [29]. Moreover, recent studies [30] have shown how the reproducibility of ^{11}C-PK11195 PET imaging is good only in large brain volumes but not in smaller subcortical regions.

6.3 Demyelination

One of the best ways to diagnose MS would be a radioligand which has myelin as its target. Unfortunately, not many compounds of this nature have been studied so far. Not many radiotracers can enter the brain and selectively bind to myelinated regions. Two of the most important radiotracers that have been tested with this purpose both in animal models and humans are (*E*,*E*)-1,4-bis(p-aminostyryl)-2-methoxybenzene (BMB) and a compound similar to BMB called case imaging compound (CIC) [31]. The study of these two compounds confirmed their non-specificity, being thus unsuitable for clinical use.

6.4 Brain metabolism

Many neurological degenerative diseases such as MS are associated with a loss of neurons, thus leading to a decrease of glucose metabolism within the brain. These are the bases on which ^{18}F-FDG-PET is used to quantitatively measure cerebral metabolic rate of glucose utilization (CMRglu), an indication of neuronal loss and the functional state of synapses [32].

There are different papers which have used ^{18}F-FDG-PET for studying MS [33, 34]. ^{18}F-FDG-PET has been used in a few studies of patients with MS. An early ^{18}F-FDG-PET study examined the relationship between the atrophy of the corpus callosum and cortical CMRglu in patients with MS and reported that corpus callosum atrophy interferes more with the left than with the right hemisphere metabolic function. ^{18}F-FDG-PET has also demonstrated that the hypometabolism of the thalamic and deep cortical gray matter structures of the temporal lobe is associated with episodic memory dysfunction in patients with MS. Moreover, the widespread reduction of CMRglu is associated with pathological performance on tests designed to assess frontal functions. Another PET study with ^{18}F-FDG has indicated hypometabolism in the frontal cortex and basal ganglia of MS patients with fatigue. Longitudinal data of CMRglu after a series of ^{18}F-FDG-PET scans have shown that cortical cerebral metabolism is significantly decreased during a two year observation period in patients with MS, suggesting a deterioration of cortical activity with disease progression. A recent study using ^{18}F-FDG-PET and magnetic resonance spectroscopy in patients with early MS has shown that reductions in cortical CMRglu are associated with reductions in cortical *N*-acetyl-aspartate/creatine in cortical and subcortical areas relevant to cognitive function.

6.5 Conclusions

Despite the encouraging results obtained so far, the full potential of PET in applications to MS is still to be realized. Currently there is a paucity of targets for molecular imaging applications in MS, and the development and validation of a wider range of relevant probes are required. PET studies targeting TSPO require replication and confirmation in a larger cohort of patients. The physiology of TSPO, and its relevance in the pathogenesis of MS, are still to be understood, and this will be important to better interpret the available data. Novel TSPO tracers can potentially have an increased sensitivity and improved accuracy of quantification, and their application will hopefully help to clarify some divergences and heterogeneity of the findings of the TSPO imaging studies in MS conducted until now. Furthermore, the effects of disease-modifying treatments on the binding of TSPO tracers have yet to be characterized. Adenosine receptor and myelin imaging are promising tools, but only pilot data have been generated so far, and a full report of their application in MS patients is not yet available. While it can be acknowledged that PET imaging is a complicated and costly process, dependent upon interdisciplinary partnerships between centers with the necessary academic expertise, financial resources and access to patients, the impact of molecular imaging on the progress of neurobiological research in MS could potentially be crucial and eventually contribute to effective clinical decision-making and patient stratification for optimization of treatment selection.

References

[1] Powers W J, Grubb R L Jr, Darriet D and Raichle M E 1985 Cerebral blood flow and cerebral metabolic rate of oxygen requirements for cerebral function and viability in humans *J. Cereb. Blood Flow Metab.* **5** 600–8

[2] Baron J C and Jones T 2012 Oxygen metabolism, oxygen extraction and positron emission tomography: historical perspective and impact on basic and clinical neuroscience *Neuroimage* **61** 492–504

[3] Abraham T and Feng J 2011 Evolution of brain imaging instrumentation *Semin. Nucl. Med.* **41** 202–19

[4] Baker W L *et al* 2011 Neurothrombectomy devices for the treatment of acute ischemic stroke: state of the evidence *Ann. Intern. Med.* **154** 243–52

[5] Furlan M, Marchal G, Viader F, Derlon J M and Baron J C 1996 Spontaneous neurological recovery after stroke and the fate of the ischemic penumbra *Ann. Neurol.* **40** 216–26

[6] Adams H, Adams R, Del Zoppo G and Goldstein L B 2005 Stroke Council of the American Heart A, American Stroke A. Guidelines for the early management of patients with ischemic stroke: 2005 guidelines update a scientific statement from the Stroke Council of the American Heart Association/American Stroke Association *Stroke* **36** 916–23

[7] Nogueira R G *et al* 2018 Thrombectomy 6 to 24 h after stroke with a mismatch between deficit and infarct *N. Engl. J. Med.* **378** 11–21

[8] Baird A E, Austin M C, McKay W J and Donnan G A 1996 Changes in cerebral tissue perfusion during the first 48 h of ischaemic stroke: relation to clinical outcome *J. Neurol. Neurosurg. Psychiatry* **61** 26–9

[9] Heiss W D 2011 The ischemic penumbra: correlates in imaging and implications for treatment of ischemic stroke. The Johann Jacob Wepfer award 2011 *Cerebrovasc. Dis.* **32** 307–20

[10] Boccardi M *et al* 2018 Assessing FDG-PET diagnostic accuracy studies to develop recommendations for clinical use in dementia *Eur. J. Nucl. Med. Mol. Imaging* **45** 1470–86

[11] Costa D C, Pilowsky L S and Ell P J 1999 Nuclear medicine in neurology and psychiatry *Lancet* **354** 1107–11

[12] Oh U *et al* 2011 Translocator protein PET imaging for glial activation in multiple sclerosis *J. Neuroimmune Pharmacol.* **6** 354–61

[13] Dheen S T, Kaur C and Ling E A 2007 Microglial activation and its implications in the brain diseases *Curr. Med. Chem.* **14** 1189–97

[14] Banati R B 2002 Visualising microglial activation *in vivo Glia* **40** 206–17

[15] Benavides J *et al* 1988 Imaging of human brain lesions with an ω3 site radioligand *Ann. Neurol.* **24** 708–12

[16] Banati R B *et al* 2000 The peripheral benzodiazepine binding site in the brain in multiple sclerosis: quantitative *in vivo* imaging of microglia as a measure of disease activity *Brain* **123** 2321–37

[17] Compston A and Coles A 2008 Multiple sclerosis *Lancet* **372** 1502–17

[18] Geurts J J and Barkhof F 2008 Grey matter pathology in multiple sclerosis *Lancet Neurol.* **7** 841–51

[19] Geurts J J, Calabrese M, Fisher E and Rudick R A 2012 Measurement and clinical effect of grey matter pathology in multiple sclerosis *Lancet Neurol.* **11** 1082–92

[20] Sormani M P 2012 Modeling the distribution of new MRI cortical lesions in multiple sclerosis longitudinal studies by Sormani M P, Calabrese M, Signori A, Giorgio A, Gallo P, de Stefano N [PLoS One 2011;6(10):E26712. Epub 2011 October 20] *Mult Scler Relat Disord.* **1** 108

[21] Tallantyre E C *et al* 2010 3 tesla and 7 tesla MRI of multiple sclerosis cortical lesions *J. Magn. Reson. Imaging* **32** 971–7

[22] Boutin H *et al* 2015 ^{18}F-GE-180: a novel TSPO radiotracer compared to ^{11}C-R-PK11195 in a preclinical model of stroke *Eur. J. Nucl. Med. Mol. Imaging* **42** 503–11

[23] Cosenza-Nashat M *et al* 2009 Expression of the translocator protein of 18 kDA by microglia, macrophages and astrocytes based on immunohistochemical localization in abnormal human brain *Neuropathol. Appl. Neurobiol.* **35** 306–28

[24] Kreutzberg G W 1996 Microglia: a sensor for pathological events in the CNS *Trends Neurosci.* **19** 312–8

[25] Kettenmann H, Hanisch U K, Noda M and Verkhratsky A 2011 Physiology of microglia *Physiol. Rev.* **91** 461–553

[26] Suzumura A, Sawada M and Marunouchi T 1996 Selective induction of interleukin-6 in mouse microglia by granulocyte-macrophage colony-stimulating factor *Brain Res.* **713** 192–8
[27] Floden A M, Li S and Combs C K 2005 Beta-amyloid-stimulated microglia induce neuron death via synergistic stimulation of tumor necrosis factor alpha and NMDA receptors *J. Neurosci.* **25** 2566–75
[28] Petit-Taboue M C *et al* 1991 Brain kinetics and specific binding of [^{11}C]PK11195 to ω3 sites in baboons: positron emission tomography study *Eur. J. Pharmacol.* **200** 347–51
[29] Boutin H *et al* 2007 *In vivo* imaging of brain lesions with [$^{(11)}$C]CLNME, a new PET radioligand of peripheral benzodiazepine receptors *Glia* **55** 1459–68
[30] Jucaite A *et al* 2012 Kinetic analysis and test–retest variability of the radioligand [^{11}C](R)-PK11195 binding to TSPO in the human brain—a PET study in control subjects *EJNMMI Res.* **2** 15
[31] Wu C, Wei J, Tian D, Feng Y, Miller R H and Wang Y 2008 Molecular probes for imaging myelinated white matter in CNS *J. Med. Chem.* **51** 6682–8
[32] Sokoloff L 1981 Localization of functional activity in the central nervous system by measurement of glucose utilization with radioactive deoxyglucose *J. Cereb. Blood Flow Metab.* **1** 7–36
[33] Pozzilli C *et al* 1992 Relationship between corpus callosum atrophy and cerebral metabolic asymmetries in multiple sclerosis *J. Neurol. Sci.* **112** 51–7
[34] Paulesu E *et al* 1996 Functional basis of memory impairment in multiple sclerosis: a [^{18}F]FDG PET study *Neuroimage* **4** 87–96

IOP Publishing

Neurological Disorders and Imaging Physics, Volume 1
Application of multiple sclerosis
Luca Saba and Jasjit S Suri

Chapter 7

Multiple sclerosis: clinical features

Gian Carlo Coghe, Giuseppe Fenu, Jessica Frau, Lorena Lorefice and Eleonora Cocco

7.1 Introduction

Multiple sclerosis (MS) is a multifaceted disease of the central nervous system (CNS) characterized by the presence of inflammatory, demyelinating and neurodegenerative processes [1, 2]. MS is a leading cause of permanent neurological disability and predominantly affects young adults in their most productive periods of life, thus representing an important socio-economic problem for individuals and society [1, 2].

The pathological hallmark of MS is the presence of demyelinating lesions spreading in the white and gray matter of the CNS (in both the brain and spinal cord) associated with axonal damage and neuronal loss. Lesions are believed to be due to the loss of tolerance regarding self-components of the CNS by the immune system with the subsequent infiltration of immune cells in the CNS and subsequent damage. The disease etiology is not completely understood, but it is considered complex and multifactorial, with interactions between genetic and environmental factors.

Generally, young adults are affected by MS, and the mean age at onset ranges between 20 and 40 years. Females are more affected, with a ratio of 2.5 to 1 compared to male individuals [3]. The onset at extreme ages is rare but is gaining attention because of its peculiar features [4–6].

Death is considered to be directly related to MS symptoms in >50% of people with MS (pwMS), while suicide and infections seem to be more prevalent with respect to the general population [7]. A recent evaluation showed a decrease in life expectancy which was determined to be 7–14 years lower than that in the general population based on previous research [7].

The course of MS disease is heterogeneous, and Lublin *et al* in 1996 [8] identified four clinical paths: relapsing–remitting (RR), secondary progressive (SP), primary progressive (PP) and progressive relapsing (PR). The majority (approximately 85%) of pwMS present an RR course that is characterized by the recurrence of clinical

doi:10.1088/2053-2563/ab1fdcch7

episodes (i.e. relapses or pousees) with highly variable symptoms lasting from a few days to some weeks or months and regressing autonomously with or without complete recovery [9]. In most pwMS, the disease changes over time, becoming progressive (SP) and leading to the accumulation of permanent disability (motor, sensitive, sphincter, cognitive, etc) in the absence of relapses. Considering the MS natural history, approximately 2%–3% of pwMS patients transition to an SP course each year. Only a minority of pwMS patients (approximately 10%–15%) present a progressive course from the beginning without relapses and are considered as PP. The last route is PR, which is rarely seen in clinical practice and is characterized by a progressive course from the onset but with the occurrence of some relapse during the disease history [8].

Typical MS progression has recently been reviewed [10], and each course has been reclassified on the basis of the presence or absence of disease activity evidenced as clinical relapses or identified by MRI. Furthermore, the progressive courses could also be defined as active if progression is observed in a given time period [7]. The first inflammatory demyelinating event suggestive of MS has been classified as 'clinically isolated syndrome' (CIS) [10]. The diagnostic criteria utilized to perform MS diagnosis have evolved over time, but they are still based on the concept of the dissemination in time (DIT) and the dissemination in space (DIS) of lesions in the CNS. However, the criteria include the possibility of satisfying DIT and DIS with clinical and/or para-clinical evidence (MRI and cerebrospinal fluid examination) and excluding other differential diagnoses (mimicking) [1, 2].

The natural history of MS has dramatically changed in recent decades due to the introduction of drugs that are able to reduce the relapse rate and disability progression. For this reason, the pharmacological therapies used in MS are defined as 'disease modified drugs' (DMD) [1, 2]. Moreover, their efficacy has improved with the introduction of more effective drugs, and the goal of the therapeutic approach has become more ambitious in the direction of 'no evidence of disease activity' (NEDA) [1, 2]. The follow-up of pwMS treated with DMD by using MRI plays an important role [1, 2].

7.2 Epidemiology

MS is widely prevalent, with approximately three million people affected worldwide. MS prevalence differs between countries (ranging between 50 and 300 per 100 000 people), and it generally follows the rule of a latitudinal gradient, because MS prevalence is higher in countries at higher latitudes and in Western countries. In particular, MS is generally present in people of Caucasian ethnicity but is unusual in Asian, Black, Native American and Maori individuals [11]. It is worth noting that the epidemiological data could be underestimated because of a lack of epidemiological studies in some large regions, such as India, China and Africa.

Many factors have been advocated as being responsible for the geographical distribution of MS as well as the different genetic representation of the *HLA-DRB1* haplotype, but some environmental factors that vary with latitude, such as a lack of sun exposure and low levels of vitamin D, are important candidates [12].

An increased MS incidence, particularly in women, has been observed in recent decades [13] with an increase in the female-to-male sex ratio. The potential role of environmental factors that primarily affect women, such as occupation, increased cigarette smoking, obesity, birth control and childbirth, is suggested by the increased incidence of MS in female individuals [14, 15].

7.3 Causes and risk factors

MS etiology is still unknown, but it is commonly believed that genetic susceptibility combined with exposure to environmental factors is required for its development [16]. Many genetic factors (each with very small effects) have been discovered in the last few years, while environmental agents are currently somewhat poorly identified.

Familial MS is estimated to be approximately 13% [17]. The recurrence risk increases with the amount of shared genetic makeup; in particular, the risk of MS occurrence in monozygotic twins is 35%, with respect to 6% in dizygotic twins and 3% in siblings [18]. MS is a multifactorial and polygenic disease, and its susceptibility is carried by polymorphisms in several genes, each with very small effects on susceptibility. Polymorphic variants in HLA class I and HLA class II genes carry the highest risk of MS [12, 18].

More than 200 gene variants have been associated with MS in genome-wide association studies; each variant exerts a small influence on MS risk, and it is plausible that different variant combinations could contribute to the disease risk in different populations and in different individuals [19]. Almost all of these variants encode molecules of the immune system, and some of them are associated with other immunomediated disorders. Notably, MS risk genes do not correspond to those found in other neurodegenerative diseases [19].

Many environmental factors have been explored [20], and most of these factors likely influence MS risk via complex gene–environment interactions acting at an individual level and in a particular time frame. Adolescence is advocated as the main period of susceptibility to environmental risk factors for MS [12]; however, there are also other delicate periods relevant for environmental factor exposure, such as pregnancy [21].

There are some well-established risk factors for MS, such as smoking, a lack of sun exposure, low vitamin D (VD) levels, early (adolescence and early adulthood) Epstein–Barr virus (EBV) infection and adolescent obesity [12].

Active smoking has been reliably demonstrated as an MS risk factor with an odds ratio (OR) of approximately 1.6 [12]. Smoking seems to influence MS risk in a dose-dependent manner. In fact, more and cumulative smoking increases the risk. Additionally, passive exposure has been associated with increased MS risk [12]. Furthermore, smoking has also been related to a quicker progression of disability and a higher risk of switching from an RRMS to an SPMS course [22]. The effect of some smoke components on promoting lung irritation from one side and the indirect systemic effects due to peribronchial lymphatic tissue on the other side could explain the association of smoke exposure with MS risk because these factors could influence immune system function [12].

The foremost determinant of VD levels is exposure to the Sun, specifically ultraviolet radiation; in fact, VD levels decrease with reduced Sun exposure, as occurs at high latitudes. VD levels have been proposed to be the main determinants in the geographical distribution of MS (latitude gradient). Numerous studies indicate an association between low VD levels and a higher risk of MS and worse outcomes (higher relapse rate MRI activity) [12]. VD in its active form (1, 25-dihydroxycholecalciferol) has an immunomodulatory effect and could influence immune tolerance mechanisms [12].

In addition, infectious diseases have been proposed as possible causes for MS occurrence. Among the various candidate pathogens, EBV is the most reliably and strongly related [23]. Notably, in epidemiological studies, up to 100% of pwMS are positive for EBV [24]. The way in which EBV could increase MS risk and influence MS occurrence is not fully understood, and one of the main hypotheses is that EBV epitopes could mimic myelin epitopes and thus molecular mimicry could lead to the origination of cross-reactive T cells and antibodies versus myelin epitopes [12].

Intriguingly, these risk factors could interact with genetic factors to induce a higher MS risk. Notably, some of these environmental factors are modifiable with changes in lifestyle; thus, preventive plans might be designed to reduce MS risk but also to influence disease outcome.

7.3.1 Neuropathology

The principal pathogenic events in MS are inflammation, demyelination, axonal loss and gliosis. These processes can be studied *in vivo* using conventional and advanced magnetic resonance imaging (MRI) [1].

Inflammation is confined in the CNS, where T and B lymphocytes are recruited by unknown antigens [25]. According to the intrinsic model, the first event occurs in the CNS, and antigens are released in the periphery. On the other hand, the extrinsic model hypothesizes that inflammation occurs outside the CNS. In both cases, in the periphery, the antigens act as triggers of the immune response, and lymphocytes enter the CNS [1].

An important feature is the aberrant activation of CD4, in particular, T helper 17 and CD8 T lymphocytes, with the insufficient function of T regulatory cells [26]. Notably, other cells also play fundamental roles in MS inflammation, and T cells are not able to affect their action without the antigen presenting cells (APC), such as B lymphocytes, microglia and dendritic cells [27]. In patients with MS, B cells release pro-inflammatory cytokines and act as APCs for the activation of T lymphocytes, with their main role being antibody independent [28]. The importance of B cells has been clear from initial studies showing the presence of oligoclonal bands in the cerebrospinal fluid in the majority of MS patients [29]. Nevertheless, many antigens and antibodies have been studied, but none of them have demonstrated a particular implication in the pathogenesis of MS [2].

Activated microglia and astrocytes also release pro-inflammatory molecules, such as chemokines, cytokines and free radicals, which can promote inflammation and neurodegeneration [30].

The characteristic demyelination is represented by focal lesions or plaques, which are localized in both the white and gray matter of the whole CNS. Three types of lesions can be distinguished in the white matter: active demyelinating, with massive presence of lymphocytes, activated microglia, macrophages and reactive astrocytes; chronic active, with macrophages mostly at the edge of the lesions; and slow expanding lesions, with activated microglia at the edge, few macrophages and transected axons. The first type is more common in relapsing patients, while the other two are observed in the SP phase. Notably, outside the focal lesions, there is the normal appearing white matter, in which both inflammation and degeneration are recognizable. In the gray matter, demyelination is commonly observed from an early period of the disease, particularly in progressive patients [2].

The progressive phase of MS is characterized by a compartmentalization of the inflammatory process in the CNS, a change from focal to diffuse damage, wide lymphocytic and monocytic infiltrates and increased cortical injury [31]. Moreover, there is more evidence of axon degeneration, astrocyte dysfunction and microglial activation. In particular, axonal loss, which also occurs in new inflammatory lesions, is slow but continuous in chronic plaques [1]. Axonal loss is associated with long-term disability, and it could be measured as brain atrophy, which is higher in patients when compared with healthy controls and could occur faster in the progressive phase and in deep gray matter [32].

Neuro- and axonal degeneration could be caused by many mechanisms, such as mitochondrial dysfunction, neuronal apoptosis, hypoxia, a pro-inflammatory environment with complement activation and cytotoxic molecules, loss of myelin trophic support, and altered glutamate homeostasis [33].

Importantly, in contrast to this damage, there is tissue repair and recovery. In fact, a restoration of nerve conduction with an attempt at remyelination could be present in demyelinated axons, but it is functionally less effective [34]. Moreover, restoration is generally limited to the edge of the lesion, and it is not observed in all MS lesions. The age of the patient, disease duration, localization of the lesions, axonal loss and presence of oligodendrocyte progenitor cells could influence the remyelination process [33], which is particularly observed in the early stages of the disease and more frequently observed in relapsing patients than in the progressive courses [35].

Additionally, cortical plasticity, with the reorganization of the cortical regions and the long-term potentiation of transmission at the synaptic level, plays an important role in the compensation of neuronal loss [36, 37].

7.4 Clinical courses

MS can be differentiated into four clinical courses: clinically isolated syndrome (CIS); relapsing–remitting (RR); secondary progressive (SP) and primary progressive (PP). The progressive relapsing (PR) phenotype was excluded from the 2013 revision as this disease course was considered vague and overlapped with other disease course subtypes [10].

- CIS is a monophasic clinical episode with symptoms and signs that reflect a demyelinating event in the CNS. The episode typically has a duration of at least 1 day, could be focal or multifocal and could develop acutely or subacutely. CIS represents an isolated attack in a patient lacking a previous history of demyelinating disease [38]. The subsequent demonstration of dissemination in space and time would lead to a diagnosis of RRMS. Natural history studies and clinical trials have shown that CIS coupled with brain MRI lesions carries a high risk of meeting the diagnostic criteria for MS [39]. The last two revisions of the MS diagnostic criteria are pushing the definition of MS to categorize a higher number of patients with a single clinical attack as MS rather than CIS [40, 41]. Typical presentation leading to a diagnosis of CIS are unilateral optic neuritis, focal supratentorial syndrome, focal brainstem or cerebellar syndrome, or partial myelopathy. Other presentations represent a red flag for alternative diagnosis and warrant further diagnostic evaluation before considering CIS: bilateral optic neuritis, complete ophthalmoplegia, complete myelopathy, encephalopathy, headache, alteration of consciousness, meningismus, or isolated fatigue [41].
- RRMS is a course characterized by relapses, with stable neurological disability between episodes. The criteria for defining a relapse are identical to those reported for CIS. During the RR course, the patient could present symptom fluctuations that are paroxysmal and do not last 24 h continuously. These symptoms must not be considered a clinical sign of focal inflammation in the CNS [38].
- SPMS. The RRMS is characterized by stable disability between clinical attacks, and the disability only lasts after a relapse by definition. However, the initial RRMS course is 'generally followed by progression with or without occasional relapses, minor remissions, and plateaus' [38]. A full year of gradual worsening of symptoms not due to superimposed relapse should be demonstrated to define an SPMS course. The evaluation is purely clinical and challenging to date, and there are no clear MRI, immunologic, or pathologic criteria to determine the transition point from RRMS to SPMS [38]. The transition is gradual and retrospectively determined, and a delay of up to 3 years was recently described [42]. This further limits the ability to study biomarkers that are able to define the transition. Several survival analyses have studied the time to SPMS in RR patients. In the Lyon and Gothenburg series, the median time was 19 years. Consistent results have been reported in other Italian and Swedish series. In the Canadian series, 30%–40% of RR patients developed SPMS within 10 years of onset. The median time to conversion was 10–15 years [42].
- PPMS. When a gradual worsening, independent of the accrual of disability over time, occurs from onset, a patient is diagnosed with PPMS [38]. Approximately 10%–15% of patients develop a PP course, which is characterized by several clinical and pathological peculiarities. Patients with worsening of disability more frequently involve motor function impairment with a pattern suggesting a myelopathy; less often, these individuals can show

progressive hemiparesis, ataxia, visual dysfunction and/or cognitive impairment [43]. The onset of progression is generally at 40–50 years. PPMS has an equal sex ratio (whereas SPMS has the same sex ratio as RRMS). However, a small proportion of MRI findings typical of MS without clinical manifestations directly convert to a PP form. Thus, PPMS is currently considered part of the MS spectrum rather than another disease [43]. However, the general consensus is that PPMS 'should remain a separate clinical course because of the absence of exacerbations prior to clinical progression, even though it likely does not have pathophysiological distinct features from SPMS' [38].

In addition to the classical phenotypes, the 2013 consensus thought that defining the ongoing disease would provide a better definition of MS for research and clinical purposes. For this reason, further categorization of MS based on clinical activity was considered in the latest classification [31]. The clinical activity is based on MRI (gadolinium-enhancing lesions or new T2 lesions) or on the clinical demonstration of CNS inflammation (clinical relapse). Moreover, even the progressive disease does not progress in a uniform fashion and stabilizes or rapidly worsens over periods. Considering these factors, both additional descriptors, namely, disease activity and progression, were considered in either the relapsing or progressive disease definition [31]. Figure 7.1 summarizes the Lublin 2013 classification.

According to this consideration, CIS and RRMS could be further subdivided into active or not active CIS and RRMS diseases. Both of the progressive (SP and PP) forms can be subdivided into active progressive disease with progression, not active

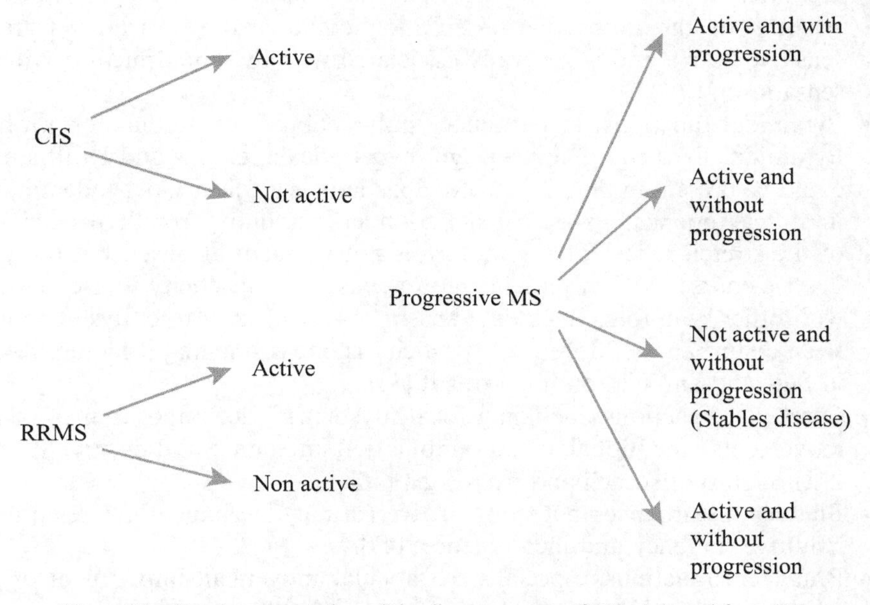

Figure 7.1. Visual representation of the disease courses of MS. Adapted from [10].

with progression, active without progression, and not active without progression. Activity must be monitored with an annual MRI scan of the brain (there are no recommendations for spinal cord scan), and progression is monitored by annual evaluation [31].

This current point of view would add a new consideration of the progressive form according the upcoming advancement in the clinical approach to the diagnosis and treatment of MS [31].

7.5 Clinical features

MS could potentially affect any part of the CNS. Correspondingly, the clinical manifestations of the disease are wide and heterogeneous. However, among the large number of possible symptoms due to MS, certain symptoms are particularly characteristic of the disease, while others are 'red flags' for reconsidering the diagnosis. This distinction is particularly relevant during the first phases of the relapsing course when the CIS diagnosis is based on a clinical presentation suggestive of inflammatory demyelination [2].

A clinical presentation evocative of MS can either singularly or contemporaneously involve several functional systems:

- The visual system, in particular optic neuritis, which is the first symptom in 25% of patients. These symptoms are characterized by a partial or total visual loss in one eye, and sometimes, dyschromatopsia and pain worsened by eye movement could also be associated [44].
- Sensory functions, including negative symptoms (deep or superficial sensation loss) or positive symptoms (paresthesia or dysesthesia). Positive symptoms are often described as tingling, 'pins and needles' feeling, tightness and swelling of the limbs. Deep sensation could lead to various degrees of sensitive ataxia and is generally associated with the impairment of vibration sensation [2].
- Pyramidal functions, in particular limb weakness or ambulation problems. Pyramidal signs (the Babinski sign, hyperreflexia, clonus and Hoffman sign) could be present in the first attack. Spasticity is a velocity-dependent increase in muscle tone with exaggerated tendon jerks resulting from hyperexcitability of the stretch reflex. This symptom is not frequent at onset, but during the disease course, 90% of patients report spasticity. Spasticity is also associated with other symptoms, including spasms, pain, urinary tract dysfunction and sleep disturbances. Moreover, spasticity is one of the major factors resulting in falls and ambulation impairment [45].
- Cerebellar functions, including focal (dysmetria, decomposition of complex movements) and global ataxia (ambulation imbalance and positive Romberg test) or slurred speech and dysphagia [46].
- Bladder disturbances both obstructive (urinary hesitancy and retention) or irritative (urgency and incontinence) [47].
- Brainstem functions, especially extraocular movement impairment or trigeminal neuralgia [2].

- Spinal cord involvement, leading to a myelitis or to a typical symptom, such as the Lhermitte sign, can be another typical presentation of MS. Lhermitte is described as an electric shock radiating down the spine or into the limbs with flexion of the neck, generally due to cervical lesions [2].
- Gait impairment is a relevant issue and a complex problem in MS. In a clinical survey of 1011 patients, La Rocca *et al* reported that 41% have walking difficulties [48]. Almost all functional systems can contribute to walking impairment (coordination, spasticity, deep sensory loss and cognition), but lifestyle, drugs and comorbidities can also affect gait [49].

Even if cognitive impairment is a clinical feature of MS in the early phase, it represents a rare onset that, similar to epileptic seizures, refers the patients to an MS clinic [2].

Neurological focal symptoms suggesting a demyelinating disease should last for ⩾24 h to be considered a relapse of MS. A clinical attack usually shows an acute or subacute evolution reaching the peak of impairment after 2 weeks and can recover completely after 2–4 weeks or last with a variable degree of disability [41]. During the RR phase, the patients could experience any of the symptoms and signs described. Moreover, the so-called invisible symptoms, such as fatigue and mood disorder, can affect a patient's quality of life [2].

The disability in MS is generally quantified by the Expanded Disability Status Scale (EDSS) introduced in 1983. The EDSS has been criticized and presents several limitations. The psychometric properties of EDSS have been deeply investigated and criticized for being insufficient; this scale addresses a broader spectrum of disabilities and demonstrates variable intra-rater reproducibility [50]. The EDSS is designed as a quantified neurological examination that considers seven functional systems (FSs): pyramidal, sensory, cerebellar, visual, brainstem, bowel/bladder and mental. Each FS subscale ranges from 0 to 5 or 0 to 6. The EDSS global score depends on single FS values plus ambulatory autonomy and ranges from 0 (no disability) to 10 (death by MS). EDSS values between 0 and 3.5 are directly determined from the FS subscales score. Global values from 4.0 to 7.0 are mostly defined by ambulation impairment, while higher values are determined by independence in activities of daily living.

EDSS is not a linear and ordinal instrument, and its inter and intra-rater variability has often been questioned. However, it is an applicable and widely used instrument. For these reasons, EDSS is considered the gold standard for evaluating MS disability [51].

7.6 Optic neuritis

Among the functional systems that could be involved in MS, the visual system is frequently affected. In fact, inflammation of the optic nerve, namely, optic neuritis (ON), represents the onset of disease in approximately 20% of patients [52]. Moreover, ON can occur during the whole course of the disease in approximately 50% of subjects with MS [53]. The typical manifestation of ON is the decline in vision in one eye over approximately one week, which is often associated with retro-orbital pain, visual field defects, and altered discrimination of colors. Partial or total resolution could occur after one month or later from the onset. The diagnosis of ON is mainly clinical, and the main tests used in general practice are acuity assessments and confrontational fields, pupillary light reflex and fundus oculi evaluations with the ophthalmoscope [54].

Nevertheless, visual evoked potentials are often performed and show a dysfunction of the optic pathways in the affected eye [55] (figure 7.2).

The visual functional system could also be affected in MS patients without episodes of ON in their lifetime, as highlighted in recent decades by the use of optical coherence tomography. This instrument is able to show the thickness of the retinal nerve fiber layer and the expression of axonal loss, if this loss is due to both previous acute inflammation, such as ON, and primary neurodegeneration [56].

7.7 Cognition

Cognitive deficits in MS involve a significant percentage of patients. Several studies have shown a prevalence between 40% and 70% of MS patients [57]. The cognitive domains principally involved in these deficits are attention, memory and executive functions [58]. Global intelligence and language are generally preserved. Dementia is rare, but cognitive impairment is a significant determinant of quality of life for MS patients [57]. Additionally, because neuropsychological assessment is difficult in daily clinical practice, the importance of cognitive impairment has increased in recent decades and represents the main concern for patients and clinicians in MS management. The use of specific diagnostic tools is necessary to detect cognitive impairment in MS. General screening instruments (i.e. the Mini Mental State Examination) are frequently associated with false negative results in MS patients.

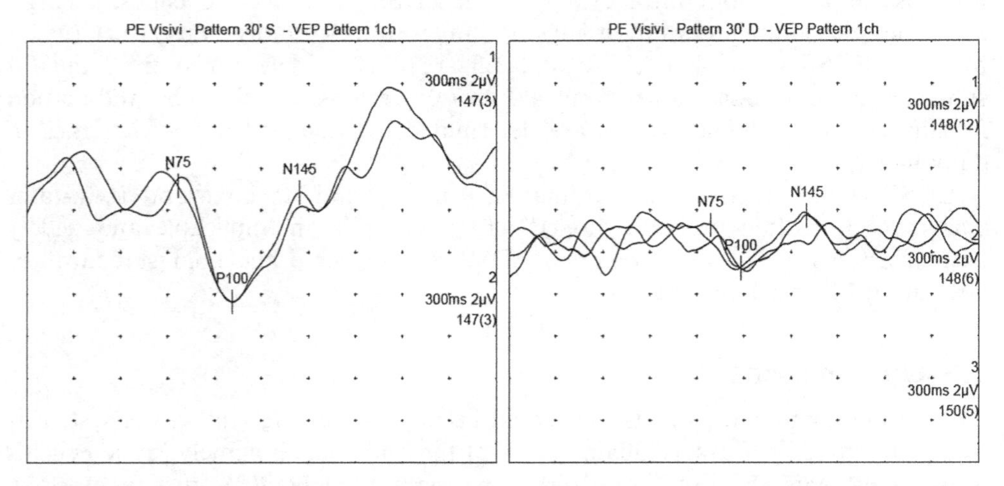

Figure 7.2. Oliclonal bands (OBs). On the left two examples of CSF without intrathecal synthesis of OBs (no OBs in the CSF or less OBs with respect to the serum). On the right two samples positive for OBs (>2 OBs in the CSF with respect to the serum).

Numerous studies have aimed to detect cognitive impairment and to characterize the possible correlations to other clinical and para-clinical features [59]. Therefore, conventional and nonconventional MRI measures have been associated with cognitive impairment in MS. A principal role has been shown for gray matter pathology (both focal lesion and volumes) and cognitive function. However, white matter lesion volume has also been detected as a strong predictor of cognitive decline in MS [9]. Several other measures have been evaluated as possibly being correlated with cognitive function in MS.

7.8 Psychiatric disorders in MS

MS is associated with a range of behavioral disorders, such as depression, bipolar affective disorder and anxiety [60]. Several epidemiological studies have reported that the lifetime prevalence of depression and anxiety in the MS population ranges from 27% to 50% [61, 62]. This variation could be due to differences in the definitions and diagnostic tools used, and the characteristics of the population studied (e.g. disease phase, level of disability) [63]. Despite the limited number of studies, a high risk of bipolar disorder was also recently reported in MS patients, with rates approaching 10% [64].

The etiology of psychiatric manifestations in MS patients is considered to be multifactorial and includes psychosocial and biological determinants, such as genetics, brain pathology and immunological changes [65]. Neuroimaging studies with advanced magnetic resonance imaging (MRI) techniques have revealed that the lesion burden in specific locations, e.g. the left arcuate fasciculus [66] and left medial inferior prefrontal cortex [60], as well as functional brain abnormalities [67], may play a causal role in depression. In addition, volumetric MRI studies have recently shown a distinctive pattern of regional atrophy in depressed patients, particularly those involving the prefrontal and temporal lobe [68] as well as subcortical structures, such as the hippocampus, nucleus caudatus and globus pallidus [69]. While white matter abnormalities, predominantly in the frontotemporal regions, have been previously reported in bipolar patients without MS [70], the radiological features of MS patients with bipolar disorder comorbidity remain unexplored.

Considering that psychiatric comorbidity is one of the main determinants of quality of life in MS patients [71], knowledge of the psychological and pathological processes related to these disorders as well as the evaluation of the relationships with MS clinical features, together with the correct diagnosis and treatment of these comorbidities, are crucial to improve the global management of MS patients.

7.9 Comorbidities in MS

The co-occurrence of other chronic medical conditions is common in MS patients [72]. Previous studies have indicated that MS is frequently associated with other autoimmune diseases, such as thyroiditis [73] and type 1 diabetes [74–76], with high rates observed in populations characteristically prone to developing autoimmune diseases, such as the Sardinian population [77]. The co-occurrence of MS with other autoimmune diseases highlights the existence of common risk factors and shared immunopathological processes [78, 79], although the heterogeneous mechanisms underlying this association remain to be clarified.

In addition, the coexistence of vascular comorbidities has also frequently been reported in subjects affected by MS, likely owing to the chronic nature of these diseases, although several MS-related conditions, such as hypomobility and obesity frequently resulting from disability, could influence this association [80, 81].

Recently, it has been hypothesized that the presence of comorbidity may explain the heterogeneity in long-term MS outcomes [80]. Both autoimmune and vascular comorbidities may have detrimental effects on the structural damage of the CNS due to their possible influence on inflammatory and neurodegenerative processes.

In line with this hypothesis, more severe nonconventional MR imaging outcomes of neurodegeneration and demyelination were reported in MS patients with co-occurring autoimmune diseases, with prevalent involvement of the gray matter and cortex [82]. Furthermore, a successive study has also documented an association between the duration of diabetes mellitus type 1 and lower brain volume measurements [83].

The impact of vascular risk comorbidities, including arterial hypertension, hyperlipidemia and diabetes mellitus types 1 and 2, on T2-lesion load, brain volumes and the volumes of deep gray matter structures (basal ganglia and thalami) was recently explored, showing lower brain volumes in early MS [84]. In addition, the co-occurrence of multiple vascular risk conditions was investigated in recent studies, indicating a significant influence, in particular on cortical gray matter volumes and longitudinal brain volume loss [85, 86].

Furthermore, a broad range of other medical chronic conditions, age-related and not age-related, of neoplastic, vascular and other natures, have frequently been reported in MS patients [87]. Thus, it is fundamental to understand the relationship between these medical conditions as well as the quantitative impact of comorbidity and its treatment on disease course, clinical/radiological features and long-term MS outcomes.

7.10 Prognosis

In addition to the risk factors, several additional factors have been evaluated as possible prognostic factors in MS [1, 2, 88].

These factors included environmental, genetic, demographic, laboratoristic, radiological and clinical features at the baseline. Prognostic factors in MS generally have been evaluated regarding the prediction of the conversion to definite clinical MS in CIS and/or to predict long-term disability accumulation. Regarding the environment and lifestyle, smoking and elevated BMI are associated with a poor prognosis; thus, at MS onset, the recommendation to avoid smoking or improve caloric intake could be helpful.

Demographic data analysis supports a better prognosis in female and younger patients. Clinical presentation with multifocal and/or motor signs and the presence of IgG oligoclonal bands in CSF are associated with poor prognosis [2]. Neuroradiological correlates of MS studies suggest that the number and volume of T2 lesions and the involvement of the infratentorial brain region or the spinal cord are associated with the worst prognosis.

In addition to the factors assessed at baseline, the influence on the prognosis of factors evaluated in the initial follow-up was examined. The factors in the early course of the disease associated with the long-term accumulation of disability are principally the relapse rate in the first 2–5 years and the occurrence of new or enlarged T2 lesions in the first year of the disease [2].

All studies regarding prognostic factors in MS have shown several limitations, principally due to the heterogeneity of the disease and the impact of the DMD administered early in the disease. These limitations represent a significant obstacle that has not allowed us to obtain natural history data concerning MS in recent decades.

7.11 Multiple sclerosis diagnosis

In recent decades, the MS diagnostic process and criteria in clinical practice have been significantly improved. Across several revisions, the diagnosis of RRMS remains based on three fundamental principles: the demonstration of DIS and DIT of the disease and the exclusion of other possible alternative diagnoses that better explain the clinical syndrome (the concept of 'No better explanation') [89, 90].

Historically, before the diffusion of the wide application of MRI for MS, the diagnosis was based on the detection of two clinical attacks to fulfill the diagnostic criteria demonstrating dissemination in time and space of the disease [89].

Improvements in the field of biomarkers have significantly modified the process to meet these principles. The increasing progress in the field of MRI has led to the integration of neuroradiological markers with an increasingly fundamental role. Since 2001, diagnostic criteria have become a combination of clinical and paraclinical parameters, initiating the era of McDonald's criteria [91].

Several revisions of the diagnostic criteria could support the clinical diagnostic process in patients with clinical demonstrations of isolated episodes of inflammatory involvement of the central nervous system [40, 41, 91, 92].

McDonald's criteria for the diagnosis of MS, first introduced in 2001 [91], with revisions in 2005 [92], 2010 [40] and 2017 [41], continue to advance. The aim of the evolution of the criteria is the need to permit an easy and early diagnosis, preserving specificity and accuracy.

The last revision of McDonald's criteria [41] permits confirmation of the diagnosis demonstrating dissemination of the disease in space and time since the first MRI scan.

The dissemination in space could be demonstrated with the presence of at least one lesion in at least two of the four CNS areas typical of MS: the cortical/juxtacortical, periventricular and infratentorial brain regions and the spinal cord (table 7.1).

The role of the cerebrospinal fluid (CSF) analysis represents the principle difference between the last revision of the diagnostic criteria compared to the previous versions. In fact, the detection of IgG oligoclonal band synthesis satisfies the criteria of dissemination in time (figure 7.3). In a patient with an MRI scan

Table 7.1. Data needed for the diagnosis of multiple sclerosis.

Clinical presentation	DIS	DIT	Diagnosis
Two clinical attacks with evidence of at least two lesions	Fulfilled	Fulfilled	Relapsing– remitting multiple sclerosis
Clinically isolated syndrome (one attack with evidence of one lesion)	⩾1 T2 lesion in at least 2 of 4 CNS areas: PV, JC/C, SC, IT or A new clinical attack i mplicating a different CNS site	Simultaneous presence of Gd+ and Gd− lesions at any time or A new T2 and/or Gd+ lesion on follow-up MRI or Presence of CSF-specific OCBs or A new clinical attack	Relapsing– remitting multiple sclerosis
Clinically isolated syndrome (one attack with evidence of at least two lesions)	Fulfilled	Simultaneous presence of Gd+ and Gd− lesions at any time or A new T2 and/or Gd+ lesion on follow-up MRI or Presence of CSF-specific OCBs or A new clinical attack	Relapsing– remitting multiple sclerosis
Two clinical attacks with evidence of one lesion	⩾1 T2 lesion in at least 2 of 4 CNS areas: PV, JC/C, SC, IT or A new clinical attack implicating a different CNS site	Fulfilled	Relapsing– remitting multiple sclerosis
One year of disability progression (retrospectively or prospectively determined) independent of clinical relapse	At least 3 of the 2 following criteria: • ⩾1 T2 lesion both in ⩾1 areas in the brain characteristic of MS (PV, JC/CL or IT) • ⩾2 T2-hyperintense lesions in the SC • Presence of CSF-specific OCBs		Primary progressive multiple sclerosis

List of abbreviations: CNS: central nervous system; PV: periventricular; JC: juxtacortical; C: cortical; IT: infratentorial; SC: spinal cord; Gd+: gadolinium-enhancing lesions; Gd−: gadolinium-non-enhancing lesions; CSF-specific OCBs: cerebrospinal fluid IgG oligoclonal bands.

satisfying DIS, the detection of intrathecal synthesis permits confirmation of the diagnosis of MS. Another difference between the last version of the diagnostic criteria and the previous version is the inclusion of the symptomatic lesion in the total count needed to meet DIS and DIT criteria and the inclusion of cortical lesions to indicate the involvement of a specific area of the CNS.

This innovation permits us to anticipate the diagnosis at the time of the first assessment in a significant percentage of patients. Several studies regarding the validation of the new criteria have confirmed these data [93, 94].

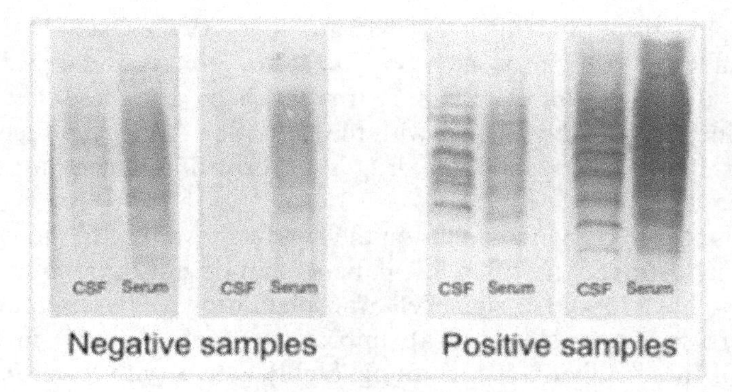

Figure 7.3. Visual evoked potential (VEP) showing a normal latency in the left eye while a latency delay and altered amplitude and morphology can be observed in the right eye. These data are suggestive of optic neuritis in the right eye.

MS diagnostic criteria should be applied only in the typical demyelinating syndromes in which these criteria have been validated [41].

For a minority of patients, clinical onset consists of a progressive worsening of the neurological disability. In these patients, the diagnosis of PPMS could be confirmed by the determination of 1 year of disability progression (retrospectively or prospectively) independent of clinical relapse and two of the following criteria: one or more T2-hyperintense lesions in at least one area in the brain characteristic of MS (periventricular, cortical and/or juxtacortical or infratentorial), two or more T2-hyperintense lesions in the spinal cord with no distinction between symptomatic or asymptomatic lesions, and demonstration of cerebrospinal fluid-specific OCBs [41].

Regarding the exclusion of other possible alternative diagnoses for both the relapsing or progressive onset of MS, some authors have proposed assessing clinical, laboratory and MRI atypical findings. These features do not rule out MS diagnosis but require additional elements to eventually confirm the diagnosis [95].

7.12 Treatments

The aims of MS treatments are three-fold:

1. To impact the disease course, reduce the relapse rate and decrease the progression of disability with DMDs.
2. To treat acute relapses.
3. To manage MS-related symptoms.

7.13 DMDs

Clinical trials have shown that DMDs are able to impact neuroinflammation and, to a lesser extent, neurodegeneration.

Until recently, all DMDs have been approved for the treatment of RR patients, and only ocrelizumab has been approved for subjects with the PP course [96].

DMDs should be started as early as possible and could be administered sequentially, according to an induction or escalation strategy. The first strategy is indicated in patients with highly active MS and involves the use of DMDs with high efficacy and a lower safety profile (second line) to obtain persistent disease remission with or without subsequent maintenance treatments by using less effective but safer drugs (first line). On the other hand, with the escalation strategy, a first-line DMD is used, and a shift versus a second-line drug is performed in unresponsive or partially responsive patients [97].

The details of DMDs, with a focus on their adverse events, are shown in table 7.2.

An important strategy useful in RR patients that do not respond to other DMDs is autologous hematopoietic stem cell transplantation. This approach is able to induce a persistent remission and an improvement of disability in RR patients, particularly if these individuals are young, highly active, with fewer prior immunotherapies and less disability [98].

Currently, due to the large number of available treatments, the choice of the correct drug at the correct time is often difficult, and both European and American guidelines have recently been developed [99, 100]. According to these guidelines, a DMD should be continued in stable patients and without safety and tolerability problems.

Older injectable DMDs, such as interferon beta and glatiramer acetate, have a lower risk of serious adverse events but also less tolerability. In contrast, with newer drugs, there is an increased risk of serious adverse events but higher tolerability [101].

In decision-making, the general safety-efficacy profile is important to consider and an individualized approach is fundamental. In fact, the risk–benefit ratio is variable between subjects and changes over time in the same person. An important issue in females is the assessment of pregnancy planning, as the majority of DMDs are contraindicated during pregnancy attempts, and only glatiramer acetate is considered safe during pregnancy [2].

7.14 Treatment of relapses

The aim of treatment is to accelerate recovery without long-term prognostic effects. Intravenous methylprednisolone at a dosage of 1000 mg for 3–5 days is the most commonly used therapy. However, high dosage oral methylprednisolone has the same efficacy. When this drug is not effective, or in patients with methylprednisolone allergies, plasma exchange and intravenous immunoglobulins are the main alternatives [1, 2].

7.15 Symptom management

A multidisciplinary approach is often mandatory for many MS-related symptoms. Both pharmacological and non-pharmacological treatments could be used, and a careful evaluation is needed. Unfortunately, the majority of drugs have no clear evidence of efficacy based on clinical trials. It is important to encourage patients to increase their level of physical activity because this approach could alleviate many MS-related symptoms [102].

Table 7.2. DMDs approved in Europe for the treatment of MS: indications and main adverse events.

Interferon beta	RRMS (*Betaferon*® also SPMS), first line	Injection site reactions Flu-like syndrome Leukopenia/thrombocytopenia Thyroid dysfunctions Transaminase increase Depression
Glatiramer acetate	RRMS, first line	Injection site reactions Panic attacks
Teriflunomide	RRMS, first line	Diarrhea Alopecia Increased blood pressure Transaminase increase
Dimethylfumarate	RRMS, first line	Flushing Gastrointestinal symptoms Lymphopenia Progressive multifocal leukoencephalopathy (PML)
Mitoxantrone	RRMS and SPMS, second line	Infections Cardiotoxicity Leukemia Fertility reduction
Natalizumab	RRMS, second line	Infections Allergic reactions Infusion-related reactions PML
Fingolimod	RRMS, second line	Infections Bradycardia Macular edema PML Skin cancer
Alemtuzumab	RRMS, second line	Infusion-related reactions Infections Autoimmune diseases
Ocrelizumab	RRMS and progressive MS, second line	Infusion-related reactions Infections Lymphopenia
Cladribine	RRMS, second line	Leukopenia Infections Alopecia

Table 7.3. Symptoms of MS and their treatments.

Fatigue	Amantadine; modafinil; acetyl-L-carnitine; physical exercise; alfacalcidol; cognitive behavioral therapy; deep transcranial magnetic stimulation
Spasticity	Baclofen; tizanidine; gabapentin; diazepam/clonazepam; nabiximols; botulinu toxin A; physical activity/physiotherapy
Ambulation dysfunction	Dalfampridine; walking aids (crutches, orthesis, walker, wheelchair)
Pain	Gabapentinoids; antidepressants; opioids; cannabinoids
Bladder dysfunction	Antimuscarinic drugs; self-catheterizations; neuromodulations; botulinum toxin A
Bowel dysfunction	Laxatives; rectal stimulants; transanal irrigation; biofeedback retraining; pelvic floor physiotherapy
Sexual dysfunction	Sildenafila; intraurethral alprostadil; pelvic floor physiotherapy; behavioral therapy
Depression	Antidepressant; cognitive behavioral therapy

A detailed description of the treatments used for the most common symptoms is shown in table 7.3.

7.16 DMD efficacy: NEDA

Combined disease-status assessments, including both clinical and MRI evaluations, are routinely used to monitor disease activity and its evolution, as well as to assess the overall effect of DMDs on disease status [103]. 'No evidence of disease activity' (NEDA), defined as the absence of clinical relapses, confirmed disability progression and MRI activity (new/enlarging T2 or T1 Gd-enhancing lesions on MRI) ('NEDA-3'), has recently been considered the treatment goal but is weighted towards inflammatory activity [104]. More recently, NEDA-4 status, including brain atrophy measurements, has also been proposed as a combined measure to capture the impact of immunotherapies on both inflammation and neurodegeneration [105] based on several studies that have correlated brain atrophy with MS long-term disability [106, 107]. However, after initiating DMDs, brain volume loss due to the effect of therapies on active focal inflammation could be observed. Therefore, to distinguish 'true' atrophy (i.e. irreversible brain tissue loss) from pseudoatrophy [108], brain volume measurements should be evaluated using rebaseline MRI images acquired after the time necessary for the drug to reach its full biological effect [109].

Another crucial point is the definition of the suboptimal response and the degree of disease activity tolerated before defining a patient as a nonresponder to a therapy. For this purpose, a scoring system based on the number of new MRI lesions, eventually in combination with clinical relapses, was proposed in patients treated with IFN-b to best predict treatment failure and guide decisions on switching treatment [110, 111]. However, a standardized algorithm to predict the response to the currently used DMDs is not yet available.

Table 7.4. MRI criteria differentiating PML from new MS lesions during natalizumab treatment.

	Multiple sclerosis	PML
Lesion size	<3 cm	>3 cm
Lesion location	Periventricular WM	Cortical GM, juxtocortical WM
Lesion appearance	Focal	Diffuse
Contrast enhancement	Infrequent during natalizumab treatment	Frequent
Lesion borders	Well-defined	Ill-defined
Other characteristics	—	Punctate T2 lesions

Abbreviation: cm: centimetres, WM: white matter, GM: gray matter.

7.17 PML risk monitoring

In recent years, the MS therapeutic armamentarium has undergone significant modifications [112]. The prolonged action of DMD drugs on the immune system, the immunosuppressive or selective action of specific drugs, and the use of therapies with different effects on the immune system could increase the risk of treatment-related infections, including CNS infections [113]. Among these infections, progressive multifocal leukoencephalopathy (PML) is a rare opportunistic infection of the CNS caused by JC virus predominantly correlated with natalizumab use, although some cases have been described with recently launched DMDs, in particular, dimethylfumarate and fingolimod [114]. Recently, a classification of PML risk of the currently available DMDs, including natalizumab in the high-risk class, dimethylfumarate and fingolimod in the low-risk class, and other DMDs in the very low- or no-risk class, has been proposed [115]. In natalizumab-treated patients, PML risk is evaluated using the new algorithm based on a duration of therapy greater than 24 months, prior immunosuppressant use, and JCV antibody positivity and index [116], and treated patients undergo PML surveillance according to FDA and EMA recommendations. In particular, it is recommended that antibody testing should be repeated every 6 months and MRI surveillance, performed using adequate protocols [117], should be adjusted if JCV is positive or if the index increases above 1.5 [118, 119]. MRI criteria differentiating PML from new MS lesions during natalizumab treatment are shown in table 7.4.

7.18 MS and quality of life

MS has a major impact on the physical, psychological and social life of patients and their families [120]. Several studies have indicated that persons with MS have lower health-related quality of life (QoL) compared to persons living with long-term conditions [121]. Several determinants of QoL have been identified in MS, including sociodemographics and disease-related variables, in particular, MS duration, clinical course and level of disability [122]. Recently, a detrimental effect on the QoL of MS patients with invisible MS symptoms, including fatigue, cognitive deficits and mood disorders, has been reported [71, 123]. Analogously, a rapidly growing body of evidence indicated that the co-occurrence of comorbidity adversely affects MS outcomes with subsequent impact on health-related daily activities [124]. Therefore, the evaluation of the determinants of QoL is complex, being influenced by multi-faceted aspects related and not related to MS. In a clinical setting, QoL is commonly measured using self-reported questionnaires; thus, the choice of tools is crucial to understanding its determinants and to assess its predictive role in health status [125]. QoL feedback to clinicians should improve interventions for the management of MS with positive effects on the long-term patient health status [126].

Finally, with a chronic illness such as MS, patients face decisions concerning treatment, multidisciplinary interventions and service availability; thus, patient engagement is particularly important for successful healthcare management [127]. Several factors, including factors related to patients, illnesses, healthcare professionals and healthcare settings, may influence the engagement of MS patients, dynamically affecting healthcare outcomes and benefits.

7.19 Conclusions

In recent decades, the world of MS management has experienced a very important change due to a better understanding of MS pathogenesis, the introduction of a large therapeutic armamentarium and the possibilities to strictly follow up the disease with the wide use of MRI.

New challenges are emerging in MS management, specifically in the search for biomarkers that could permit the prediction of the evolution of the disease in a single person and allow for a personalized approach to the disease.

References

[1] Thompson A J, Baranzini S, Geurts J, Hemmer B and Ciccarelli O 2018 Multiple sclerosis *Lancet* **391** 1622–36

[2] Filippi M *et al* 2018 Multiple sclerosis *Nat. Rev. Dis. Primers* **4** 49

[3] Greer J M and McCombe P A 2011 Role of gender in multiple sclerosis: clinical effects and potential molecular mechanisms *J. Neuroimmunol.* **234** 7–18

[4] Krupp L B *et al* 2013 International Pediatric Multiple Sclerosis Study Group criteria for pediatric multiple sclerosis and immune-mediated central nervous system demyelinating disorders: revisions to the 2007 definitions *Mult. Scler.* **19** 1261–7

[5] Yeshokumar A K, Narula S and Banwell B 2017 Pediatric multiple sclerosis *Curr. Opin. Neurol.* **30** 216–21

[6] Bermel R A, Rae-Grant A D and Fox R J 2010 Diagnosing multiple sclerosis at a later age: more than just progressive myelopathy *Mult. Scler.* **16** 1335–40

[7] Scalfari A *et al* 2013 Mortality in patients with multiple sclerosis *Neurology* **81** 184–92

[8] Lublin F D and Reingold S C 1996 Defining the clinical course of multiple sclerosis: results of an international survey *Neurology* **46** 907–11

[9] McDonald W I 2000 Relapse, remission, and progression in multiple sclerosis *N. Engl. J. Med.* **343** 1486–7

[10] Lublin F D *et al* 2014 Defining the clinical course of multiple sclerosis: the 2013 revisions *Neurology* **83** 278–86

[11] Rosati G 2001 The prevalence of multiple sclerosis in the world: an update *Neurol. Sci.* **22** 117–39
[12] Olsson T, Barcellos L F and Alfredsson L 2017 Interactions between genetic, lifestyle and environmental risk factors for multiple sclerosis *Nat. Rev. Neurol.* **13** 25–36
[13] Alonso A and Hernan M A 2008 Temporal trends in the incidence of multiple sclerosis: a systematic review *Neurology* **71** 129–35
[14] Koch-Henriksen N and Sorensen P S 2010 The changing demographic pattern of multiple sclerosis epidemiology *Lancet Neurol.* **9** 520–32
[15] Orton S M *et al* 2006 Sex ratio of multiple sclerosis in Canada: a longitudinal study *Lancet Neurol.* **5** 932–6
[16] Compston A and Coles A 2008 Multiple sclerosis *Lancet* **372** 1502–17
[17] Harirchian M H *et al* 2017 Worldwide prevalence of familial multiple sclerosis: a systematic review and meta-analysis *Mult. Scler. Relat. Disord.* **20** 43–7
[18] Compston A and Coles A 2002 Multiple sclerosis *Lancet* **359** 1221–31
[19] Cotsapas C and Mitrovic M 2018 Genome-wide association studies of multiple sclerosis *Clin. Transl. Immunol.* **7** e1018
[20] Simpson S Jr *et al* 2011 Latitude is significantly associated with the prevalence of multiple sclerosis: a meta-analysis *J. Neurol. Neurosurg. Psychiatry* **82** 1132–41
[21] Mirzaei F *et al* 2011 Gestational vitamin D and the risk of multiple sclerosis in offspring *Ann. Neurol.* **70** 30–40
[22] Healy B C *et al* 2009 Smoking and disease progression in multiple sclerosis *Arch. Neurol.* **66** 858–64
[23] Endriz J, Ho P P and Steinman L 2017 Time correlation between mononucleosis and initial symptoms of MS *Neurol. Neuroimmunol. Neuroinflamm.* **4** e308
[24] Haahr S *et al* 2004 A role of late Epstein–Barr virus infection in multiple sclerosis *Acta Neurol. Scand.* **109** 270–5
[25] Schirmer L, Srivastava R and Hemmer B 2014 To look for a needle in a haystack: the search for autoantibodies in multiple sclerosis *Mult. Scler.* **20** 271–9
[26] Baecher-Allan C, Kaskow B J and Weiner H L 2018 Multiple sclerosis: mechanisms and immunotherapy *Neuron* **97** 742–68
[27] Jelcic I *et al* 2018 Memory B cells activate brain-homing, autoreactive CD4+ T cells in multiple sclerosis *Cell* **175** 85–100
[28] Li R, Patterson K and Bar-Or A 2018 Reassessing the contributions of B cells in multiple sclerosis *Nat. Rev. Immunol.* **19** 696–707
[29] Kabat E A, Glusman M and Knaub V 1948 Immunochemical estimation of albumin and gamma globulin in normal and pathological cerebrospinal fluid *Fed. Proc.* **7** 306
[30] Dendrou C A, Fugger L and Friese M A 2015 Immunopathology of multiple sclerosis *Nat. Rev. Immunol.* **15** 545–58
[31] Kutzelnigg A *et al* 2005 Cortical demyelination and diffuse white matter injury in multiple sclerosis *Brain* **128** 2705–12
[32] Eshaghi A *et al* 2018 Deep grey matter volume loss drives disability worsening in multiple sclerosis *Ann. Neurol.* **83** 210–22
[33] Lassmann H 2018 Multiple sclerosis pathology *Cold Spring Harb. Perspect. Med.* **8** a028936
[34] Franklin R J and Ffrench-Constant C 2008 Remyelination in the CNS: from biology to therapy *Nat. Rev. Neurosci.* **9** 839–55

[35] Goldschmidt T *et al* 2009 Remyelination capacity of the MS brain decreases with disease chronicity *Neurology* **72** 1914–21
[36] Tomassini V *et al* 2012 Neuroplasticity and functional recovery in multiple sclerosis *Nat. Rev. Neurol.* **8** 635–46
[37] Weiss S *et al* 2014 Disability in multiple sclerosis: when synaptic long-term potentiation fails *Neurosci. Biobehav. Rev.* **43** 88–99
[38] Miller D *et al* 2005 Clinically isolated syndromes suggestive of multiple sclerosis, part I: natural history, pathogenesis, diagnosis, and prognosis *Lancet Neurol.* **5** 281–8
[39] O'Riordan J I *et al* 1998 The prognostic value of brain MRI in clinically isolated syndromes of the CNS. A 10-year follow-up *Brain* **121** 495–503
[40] Polman C H *et al* 2011 Diagnostic criteria for multiple sclerosis: 2010 revisions to the McDonald criteria *Ann. Neurol.* **69** 292–302
[41] Thompson A J *et al* 2018 Diagnosis of multiple sclerosis: 2017 revisions of the McDonald criteria *Lancet Neurol.* **17** 162–73
[42] Rovaris M *et al* 2006 Secondary progressive multiple sclerosis: current knowledge and future challenges *Lancet Neurol.* **5** 343–54
[43] Ontaneda D *et al* 2017 Progressive multiple sclerosis: prospects for disease therapy, repair, and restoration of function *Lancet* **389** 1357–66
[44] Toosy A T, Deborah F, Mason D F and Miller D H 2014 Optic neuritis *Lancet Neurol.* **13** 83–99
[45] McAlpine D 1972 *Multiple Sclerosis: A Reappraisal* 2nd edn ed D McAlpine, C E Lumsden and E D Acheson (London: Churchill Livingstone) pp 132–96
[46] Parmar K *et al* 2018 The role of the cerebellum in multiple sclerosis—150 years after Charcot *Neurosci. Biobehav. Rev.* **89** 85–98
[47] Ghezzi A E *et al* 2016 Diagnostic tools for assessment of urinary dysfunction in MS patients without urinary disturbances *Neurol. Sci.* **37** 437–42
[48] LaRocca N G 2011 Impact of walking impairment in multiple sclerosis *Patient Relat. Outcome Meas.* **4** 189–201
[49] Bethoux F 2003 Gait disorders in multiple sclerosis *Continuum* **19** 1007–22
[50] Hobart J, Freeman J and Thompson A 2000 Kurtzke scales revisited: the application of psychometric methods to clinical intuition *Brain* **123** 1027–40
[51] Goodkin D E 1992 Inter and intrarater scoring greement using grades 1.0 to 3.5 of Kurtzke EDSS. Multiple Sclerosis Collaborative Research Group *Neurology* **42** 859–63
[52] Petzold A *et al* 2014 The investigation of acute optic neuritis: a review and proposed protocol *Nat. Rev. Neurol.* **10** 447–58
[53] Optic Neuritis Study Group 2008 Multiple sclerosis risk after optic neuritis *Arch. Neurol.* **65** 727–32
[54] Frohman E M *et al* 2005 The neuro-ophthalmology of multiple sclerosis *Lancet Neurol.* **4** 111–21
[55] Hood D C, Odel J G and Winn B J 2003 The multifocal visual evoked potential *J Neuro-Ophthalmol.* **23** 279–89
[56] Parisi V *et al* 1999 Correlation between morphological and functional retinal impairment in multiple sclerosis patients *Invest. Ophthalmol. Vis. Sci.* **40** 2520–27
[57] Chiaravalloti N D and DeLuca J 2008 Cognitive impairment in multiple sclerosis *Lancet Neurol.* **7** 1139–51

[58] Sumowski J F *et al* 2018 Cognition in multiple sclerosis: state of the field and priorities for the future *Neurology* **90** 278–88

[59] Rocca M A *et al* 2015 Clinical and imaging assessment of cognitive dysfunction in multiple sclerosis *Lancet Neurol.* **14** 302–17

[60] Feinstein A *et al* 2013 Cognitive and neuropsychiatric disease manifestations in MS *Mult. Scler. Relat. Disord.* **2** 4–12

[61] Patten S B *et al* 2003 Major depression in multiple sclerosis: a population-based perspective *Neurology* **61** 1524–7

[62] Sadovnick A D *et al* 1996 Depression and multiple sclerosis *Neurology* **46** 628–32

[63] Boeschoten R E *et al* 2017 Prevalence of depression and anxiety in multiple sclerosis: a systematic review and meta-analysis *J. Neurol. Sci.* **372** 331–41

[64] Carta M G *et al* 2014 The risk of bipolar disorders in multiple sclerosis *J. Affect. Disord.* **155** 255–60

[65] Feinstein A *et al* 2014 The link between multiple sclerosis and depression *Nat. Rev. Neurol.* **10** 507–17

[66] Pujol J *et al* 1997 Lesions in the left arcuate fasciculus region and depressive symptoms in multiple sclerosis *Neurology* **49** 1105–10

[67] Bonavita S *et al* 2017 Default mode network changes in multiple sclerosis: a link between depression and cognitive impairment? *Eur. J. Neurol.* **24** 27–36

[68] Pravatà E *et al* 2017 Gray matter trophism, cognitive impairment, and depression in patients with multiple sclerosis *Mult. Scler.* **23** 1864–74

[69] Stuke H *et al* 2016 Cross-sectional and longitudinal relationships between depressive symptoms and brain atrophy in MS patients *Front. Hum. Neurosci.* **10** 622

[70] Bruno S, Cercignani M and Ron M A 2008 White matter abnormalities in bipolar disorder: a voxel-based diffusion tensor imaging study *Bipolar Disord.* **10** 460–8

[71] Carta M G *et al* 2014 Multiple sclerosis and bipolar disorders: the burden of comorbidity and its consequences on quality of life *J. Affect. Disord.* **167** 192–7

[72] Marrie R A 2016 Comorbidity in multiple sclerosis: some answers, more questions *Int. J. MS Care* **18** 271–2

[73] Karni A and Abramsky O 1999 Association of MS with thyroid disorders *Neurology* **53** 883–5

[74] Dorman J S *et al* 2003 Type 1 diabetes and multiple sclerosis: together at last *Diabetes Care* **26** 3192–3

[75] Nielsen N M *et al* 2006 Type 1 diabetes and multiple sclerosis: a Danish population-based cohort study *Arch. Neurol.* **63** 1001–4

[76] Hussein W I and Reddy S S 2006 Prevalence of diabetes in patients with multiple sclerosis *Diabetes Care* **29** 1984–5

[77] Marrosu M G *et al* 2002 Patients with multiple sclerosis and risk of type 1 diabetes mellitus in Sardinia, Italy: a cohort study *Lancet* **359** 1461–5

[78] Stinissen P, Raus J and Zhang J 1997 Autoimmune pathogenesis of multiple sclerosis: role of autoreactive T lymphocytes and new immunotherapeutic strategies *Crit. Rev. Immunol.* **17** 33–75

[79] Steri M *et al* 2017 Overexpression of the cytokine BAFF and autoimmunity risk *N. Engl. J. Med.* **376** 1615–26

[80] Marrie R A *et al* 2016 Differing trends in the incidence of vascular comorbidity in MS and the general population *Neurol. Clin. Pract.* **6** 120–8

[81] Tettey P *et al* 2014 Vascular comorbidities in the onset and progression of multiple sclerosis *J. Neurol. Sci.* **347** 23–33
[82] Zivadinov R *et al* 2016 Autoimmune comorbidities are associated with brain injury in multiple sclerosis *AJNR Am. J. Neuroradiol.* **37** 1010–6
[83] Lorefice L *et al* 2018 Autoimmune comorbidities in multiple sclerosis: what is the influence on brain volumes? A case-control MRI study *J. Neurol.* **265** 1096–101
[84] Pichler A *et al* 2017 The impact of vascular risk factors on brain volume and lesion load in patients with early multiple sclerosis *Mult. Scler.* **25** 48–54
[85] Jakimovski D *et al* 2018 Hypertension and heart disease are associated with development of brain atrophy in multiple sclerosis: a 5-year longitudinal study *Eur. J. Neurol.* **26** 87-e8
[86] Lorefice L *et al* 2018 Assessing the burden of vascular risk factors on brain atrophy in multiple sclerosis: a case-control MRI study *Mult. Scler. Relat. Disord.* **27** 74–8
[87] Edwards L J and Constantinescu C S 2004 A prospective study of conditions associated with multiple sclerosis in a cohort of 658 consecutive outpatients attending a multiple sclerosis clinic *Mult. Scler.* **10** 575–81
[88] Dobson R and Giovannoni G 2018 Multiple sclerosis—a review *Eur. J. Neurol.* **26** 27–40
[89] De Angelis F *et al* 2018 New MS diagnostic criteria in practice *Pract. Neurol.* **19** 64–7
[90] Charil A *et al* 2006 MRI and the diagnosis of multiple sclerosis: expanding the concept of 'no better explanation' *Lancet Neurol.* **5** 841–52
[91] McDonald W I *et al* 2001 Recommended diagnostic criteria for multiple sclerosis: guidelines from the International Panel on the Diagnosis of Multiple Sclerosis *Ann. Neurol.* **50** 121–7
[92] Polman C H *et al* 2005 Diagnostic criteria for multiple sclerosis: 2005 revisions to the 'McDonald Criteria' *Ann. Neurol.* **58** 840–6
[93] Gaetani L *et al* 2018 2017 revisions of McDonald criteria shorten the time to diagnosis of multiple sclerosis in clinically isolated syndromes *J. Neurol.* **265** 2684–7
[94] van der Vuurst de Vries R M *et al* 2018 Application of the 2017 revised McDonald criteria for multiple sclerosis to patients with a typical clinically isolated syndrome *JAMA Neurol.* **75** 1392–8
[95] Solomon A J, Naismith R T and Cross A H 2018 Misdiagnosis of multiple sclerosis: impact of the 2017 McDonald criteria on clinical practice *Neurology* **92** 26–33
[96] Montalban X *et al* 2017 Ocrelizumab versus placebo in primary progressive multiple sclerosis *N. Engl. J. Med.* **376** 209–20
[97] Fenu G *et al* 2015 Induction and escalation therapies in multiple sclerosis *Antiinflamm. Antiallergy Agents Med. Chem.* **14** 26–34
[98] Muraro P A *et al* 2017 Long-term outcomes after autologous hematopoietic stem cell transplantation for multiple sclerosis *JAMA Neurol.* **74** 459–69
[99] Montalban X *et al* 2018 ECTRIMS/EAN guidelines on the pharmacological treatment of people with multiple sclerosis *Mult. Scler.* **24** 96–120
[100] Rae-Grant A *et al* 2018 Practice guideline recommendations summary: disease-modifying therapies for adults with multiple sclerosis *Neurology* **90** 777–88
[101] Comi G, Radaelli M and Soelberg Sorensen P 2017 Evolving concepts in the treatment of relapsing multiple sclerosis *Lancet* **389** 1347–56
[102] Motl R W *et al* 2017 Exercise in patients with multiple sclerosis *Lancet Neurol.* **16** 848–56
[103] Bevan C J and Cree B A 2014 Disease activity free status: a new end point for a new era in multiple sclerosis clinical research? *JAMA Neurol.* **71** 269–70

[104] Giovannoni G *et al* 2015 Is it time to target no evident disease activity (NEDA) in multiple sclerosis? *Mult. Scler. Relat. Disord.* **4** 329–33

[105] Kappos L *et al* 2016 Inclusion of brain volume loss in a revised measure of 'no evidence of disease activity' (NEDA-4) in relapsing-remitting multiple sclerosis *Mult. Scler.* **22** 1297–305

[106] Popescu V, Agosta F and Hulst H E 2013 Brain atrophy and lesion load predict long term disability in multiple sclerosis *J. Neurol. Neurosurg. Psychiatry* **84** 1082–91

[107] De Stefano N *et al* 2018 Reduced brain atrophy rates are associated with lower risk of disability progression in patients with relapsing multiple sclerosis treated with cladribine tablets *Mult. Scler.* **24** 222–26

[108] De Stefano N and Arnold D L 2015 Towards a better understanding of pseudoatrophy in the brain of multiple sclerosis patients *Mult. Scler.* **21** 675–6

[109] Freedman M S *et al* 2013 Treatment optimization in MS: Canadian MS Working Group updated recommendations *Can. J. Neurol. Sci.* **40** 307–23

[110] Sormani M P *et al* 2013 Scoring treatment response in patients with relapsing multiple sclerosis *Mult. Scler.* **19** 605–12

[111] Sormani M P *et al* 2016 Assessing response to interferon-β in a multicenter dataset of patients with MS *Neurology* **87** 134–40

[112] Chitnis T, Giovannoni G and Trojano M 2018 Complexity of MS management in the current treatment era *Neurology* **90** 761–2

[113] Grebenciucova E and Pruitt A 2017 Infections in patients receiving multiple sclerosis disease-modifying therapies *Curr. Neurol. Neurosci. Rep.* **17** 88

[114] Zaheer F and Berger J R 2012 Treatment-related progressive multifocal leukoencephalopathy: current understanding and future steps *Ther. Adv. Drug Saf.* **3** 227–39

[115] Berger J R 2017 Classifying PML risk with disease modifying therapies *Mult. Scler. Relat. Disord.* **12** 59–63

[116] Schwab N *et al* 2017 Natalizumab-associated PML: challenges with incidence, resulting risk, and risk stratification *Neurology* **88** 1197–205

[117] McGuigan C *et al* 2016 Stratification and monitoring of natalizumab associated progressive multifocal leukoencephalopathy risk: recommendations from an expert group *J. Neurol. Neurosurg. Psychiatry* **87** 117–25

[118] Igra M S *et al* 2017 Multiple sclerosis update: use of MRI for early diagnosis, disease monitoring and assessment of treatment related complications *Br. J. Radiol.* **90** 20160721

[119] Wattjes M P *et al* 2018 Inflammatory natalizumab-associated PML: baseline characteristics, lesion evolution and relation with PML-IRIS *J. Neurol. Neurosurg. Psychiatry* **89** 535–41

[120] Uccelli M M 2014 The impact of multiple sclerosis on family members: a review of the literature *Neurodegener. Dis. Manag.* **4** 177–85

[121] Riazi A *et al* 2003 Using the SF-36 measure to compare the health impact of multiple sclerosis and Parkinson's disease with normal population health profiles *J. Neurol. Neurosurg. Psychiatry* **74** 710–14

[122] Tacchino A, Brichetto G, Zaratin P, Battaglia M A and Ponzio M 2018 Self-assessment reliability in multiple sclerosis: the role of socio-demographic, clinical, and quality of life aspects *Neurol. Sci.* **40** 617–20

[123] Mitchell A J *et al* 2005 Quality of life and its assessment in multiple sclerosis: integrating physical and psychological components of wellbeing *Lancet Neurol.* **4** 556–66

[124] Marrie R A 2017 Comorbidity in multiple sclerosis: implications for patient care *Nat. Rev. Neurol.* **13** 375–82

[125] Baumstarck K *et al* 2013 Measuring the quality of life in patients with multiple sclerosis in clinical practice: a necessary challenge *Mult. Scler. Int.* **2013** 524894

[126] Solari A 2005 Role of health-related quality of life measures in the routine care of people with multiple sclerosis *Health Qual. Life Outcomes* **3** 16

[127] Rieckmann P *et al* 2015 Achieving patient engagement in multiple sclerosis: a perspective from the multiple sclerosis in the 21st Century Steering Group *Mult. Scler. Relat. Disord.* **4** 202–18

IOP Publishing

Neurological Disorders and Imaging Physics, Volume 1
Application of multiple sclerosis
Luca Saba and Jasjit S Suri

Chapter 8

Volumetric analysis and atrophy in multiple sclerosis

Francesco Destro, Jasjit S Suri and Luca Saba

8.1 Brain atrophy

Brain atrophy is a term that generally describes cerebral tissue loss that can be attributed to the loss of axons, myelin or glial cells. Also blood, tissue fluids and blood vessels contribute to the definition of a brain volume. In neuroradiological examinations, such as brain CT or MRI, atrophy is a frequent finding and is frequently described. Cerebral tissue loss could be paraphysiological evidence or could be related to many pathologies. Despite the radiologist generally reporting it as aspecific, it is important to describe volume loss qualitatively and to quantify it, because in some diseases it is a fundamental parameter for the patient prognosis. It is important to describe if the tissue loss is generalized or localized to specific brain areas, for example temporo-mesial, basal ganglia or cerebellar atrophy, which can be a specific sign of a specific disease. It is also important to know the patient history to identify a specific kind of atrophy, for example related to a tissue loss after an ischemic or a demyelinating event.

8.2 Conditions associated with brain atrophy

Focal atrophy is frequently an age related finding or can be found in patients suffering from cerebrovascular disease or end-stage multiple sclerosis, or certain neurodegenerative diseases such as progressive sopra-nuclear palsy. In contrast, generalized atrophy can be observed in post-traumatic or post-ischemic injuries, Alzheimer's or Parkinson's disease, frontotemporal dementia and Huntington's disease.

doi:10.1088/2053-2563/ab1fdcch8

8.3 Qualitative imaging findings related to brain volume reduction

Traditionally, the fast method for evaluating cerebral atrophy, particularly in patients suffering from dementias, is visual rating scales. The most used is the scale for global cortical atrophy which allows us to categorize patients into four different cortical atrophy stages, based on the size of the sulci and on the thickness of the cortical gyri in FLAIR images. To evaluate localized atrophy of the temporal lobe, as in patients with suspected Alzheimer's disease, sometimes the medial temporal lobe atrophy (MTA-)score is used, based on the width of the choroid fissure and the temporal horn and the height of the hippocampal formation. For the evaluation of AD or other dementias, the MTA scale shows good accuracy for diagnosis and follow up, and is supported by volumetric studies *in vivo* and post-mortem data. A final example of a visual rating scale frequently used in the radiological evaluation of neurodegeneration processes is the Fazekas scale, a useful and rapid method to establish the periventricular, age and vascular related periventricular and deep white matter hyperintensities classified by their shape, number and confluence. For MS these visual rating scales, which evaluate coarse brain tissue losses, often in advanced stages of disease, are not useful. A more objective and precise method to quantitatively establish minimal tissue losses is needed to establish the progression of the disease, the efficacy of treatment and the prognosis for patients.

8.4 Pathological bases of atrophy in MS

8.4.1 White matter demyelination pathogenesis

Multiple sclerosis is classically described as a disease of cerebral white matter. The pathologic basis of myelin loss is an immune mediated inflammatory reaction against oligodendrocyte and myelin sheets. The main stages described in the pathogenesis of multiple sclerosis are an increased expression of adhesion molecules by activated endothelial cells, disruption of the blood–brain barrier, transendothelial migration of activated CD4+ T lymphocytes and macrophages into the CNS, and development of multifocal demyelinating lesions. The classical idea that MS is a pathologic process that involves only white matter was recently revised, due to the observation of the involvement of gray matter from the first stages of the disease [1]. Thus both gray and white matter of the optic nerves, cerebral hemispheres, brain stem and spinal cord are involved. The main histological findings of the MS acute demyelinating plaques reveal inflammatory infiltrates composed of lymphocytes and macrophages, sharply demarcated areas of myelin loss and astrocytic proliferation. During disease progression the inflammation infiltrates decrease while the neuro-degenerative mechanism becomes predominant. In this stage, the patient's disability progresses and there is a reduced response to available immunotherapies [2].

At the end of the inflammatory cascade, sustained by T CD+ lymphocytes, activated macrophages and microglia are the main protagonists of the axonal damage and the subsequent brain atrophy. Cytotoxic and trophic factors are secreted by these cells to destroy axons and to phagocyte myelin debris. Indeed, one of the major consequences of the inflammatory cascade at the initial stage is the axonal damage, the severity of which correlates with the inflammatory activity [2].

8.4.2 Gray matter degeneration in MS

As in other chronic diseases of the central nervous system (CNS), such as Alzheimer's, Parkinson's and amyotrophic lateral sclerosis, neurodegeneration is a main feature of MS disease progression, and brain atrophy is the macroscopically and radiologically detectable finding that is associated. Reversible and irreversible neurodegeneration cannot be attributed only to the late stage of the disease, as recently it has been demonstrated that axon loss occurs at early stages of the disease. Moreover, the grade of axonal loss or brain atrophy longitudinally correlates with the grade of disability [3–5]. There is a discrepancy between the stereological analysis of neuronal death and quantitative gray matter volumes identified by MRI, and this could be explained by the neuron surface distributed on the neurons being vastly greater than that on the cell soma [6].

Axons are relatively fragile cells and can easily be damaged by traumatic, ischemic, oxidative and inflammatory insults. In MS disease neurons are more prone to degeneration because of myelin loss, which causes an increasing energy demand for signal conduction with reduced energy supply [6]. Additionally, oligodendrocyte dysfunction causes a loss of the trophic functions of the neural cell.

The main histopathologic feature of axonal death is the spheroid and vesicular aspect which reflects impaired axonal transport. The failure of neuronal intracellular transport is also reflected by immune histochemical studies, where an abnormal stack of amyloid precursor protein (APP) is marked by the antibody. Other proof of impaired axonal transport in MS patient lesions is the presence of the neurofilament heavy chain in a non-phosphorylated isoform, whereas the phosphorylated form is abundant in normal axons [7].

Another common feature of MS neurodegeneration is the frequent presence of transacted axons. Iron deposition, linked to inflammatory processes, may be a cause of neuronal degeneration. Many studies demonstrate, by the use of T2* MRI sequences, that there is a major deposition of this paramagnetic element in inflammatory plaques. Iron could directly generate oxidative stress and irreversibly damage neurons [2].

The oxidative stress caused by the pathology is also documented by MRI spectroscopy, which shows a high presence of *N*-acetyl-aspartate (NAA), a biochemical marker of the mitochondrial activity of normal neurons. Low levels of NAA could be attributed to impaired mitochondrial activity due to oxidative stress or neural loss. Decreased NAA levels are found in normal apparent white matter (NAWM) in multiple sclerosis in early stages of the disease [2] and this could demonstrate axonal loss even in the early stages of the disease.

Also, the inferred axonal transport mechanisms could be related to neuronal cell death in MS, and this is well demonstrated in immuno-histological studies, where a high grade of accumulation of APP is shown in swollen areas of injured axons. In these areas there is also an increase of expression of high grade voltage calcium channels and this could cause an increased influx of calcium ions and an activation of caspase mediated apoptosis [2].

Finally, free glutamate, which can be increased in the inflammatory events of MS, is linked to an increase of cellular death, due to its high activation of glutamate receptors and high grade of excitotoxicity. The contribution of glial cell proliferation in MS patients is less than that of myelin and axons and is balanced by oligodendrocyte loss.

Indeed, changes in tissue fluids can have an important effect on brain volumes and inflammatory stages where there are areas of active inflammation and vasogenic edema can increase brain volumes. The main feature of axonal damage is that the distal and proximal tract of the cell are also involved in the cell death. It involves other cells that are not directly injured and which are distant from the insult, and this is called transneuronal degeneration, and that rarely could be find a sort of regeneration. Classically, three different kinds of neuronal degeneration are described: anterograde trans-synaptic degeneration, retrograde degeneration and Wallerian degeneration [6]. Anterograde degeneration is the classic mechanism of optic nerve death and is described as a trans-synaptic death that occurs for neurons that are not directly injured that receive synaptic input from injured neurons. This mechanism of neurodegeneration of the cortico-spinal tract lacks evidence in MS pathology [6]. Retrograde degeneration is a kind of neurodegeneration that starts distally at the site of the axonal lesion and propagates backwards towards the cell body, leading to cell death. In MS the presence of axonal lesions could be the cause of cortical neuron death. Wallerian degeneration consists in the degeneration of the axon below the axonal lesion and is a possible mechanism of volume loss in MS neurodegeneration, although there is lack of evidence [6].

8.5 Neurodegeneration and MS, clinical implications

Axonal loss is the major determinant of neurological disability in MS. The axonal loss in the first stages of the disease is balanced by the response of the oligodendrocyte to myelin loss. Axonal loss begins at disease onset and correlates with the degree of inflammation. Axonal loss remains silent in the early stages of the disease because of the compensatory resources of other neurons. After a certain threshold axonal loss becomes clinically relevant.

8.6 Brain volumes and how to calculate them

The methods used to study the tissue volumes should be reproducible, sensitive to change, accurate and practical to implement.

Data acquisition. Spatial and contrast resolution are essential for a good quantification of brain volumes. In the past, axial 2D scans were used, but the possibility of having high resolution images and re-slicing datasets makes 3D acquisitions, defined by isotropic voxels $1 \times 1 \times 1$ with multiple image contrasts, more appropriate for these kinds of studies [8]. Moreover, the need to have high contrast resolution, makes the use of the GRE echo sequences and the IR sequences, where there is suppression of the CSF fluids, mandatory [8]. 3D acquisition is preferred because of the possibility of patient motion during other types of acquisitions, which can cause errors in estimating volumes, and also the acquisition between two time-points will inevitably introduce interpolation artifacts.

Data analysis methods. An experienced observer is required who is confident in identifying the normal radiological neuroanatomy and the pathologic appearance of CNS pathologies. Both gray and white matter could be segmented. Outlining brain tissue with manual segmentation is easy and the software for these kinds of evaluations is easy to find, but it is very time-consuming and can present great intra- and inter-observer variability, which reduces the accuracy and reproducibility, so semi-automatic or completely automatic software is advisable. Automated segmentation provides good reproducibility and is time saving. It can also verify the spatial resolutions.

8.7 Linear and regional measures

Linear measures are the simplest way to estimate brain atrophy in MS, because they can be applied to various sequences, and also 2D images. The most commonly applied linear measurement is the brain width on axial images, based on the principle that ventricular enlargement results in small brain tissue loss.

8.8 Segmentation based brain volume measurement methods

Segmentation techniques are useful post-processing methods that are commonly used for measuring and visualizing different brain structures, for delineating lesions, for analysis of brain development, and for image guided interventions and surgical planning.

The segmentation of an MRI scan is based on the concept of the image element, which is a pixel in 2D images, defined by two spatial coordinates, and the voxels of 3D images are defined by three spatial coordinates. To every voxel or pixel is assigned a value based on the tissue resonance signal. The spatial characteristic of the image element defines the spatial resolution of the image: the smallest is the voxel, the highest is the spatial resolution. In the image matrix, which is composed of a various number of pixels or voxels, segmentation can divide this into areas of elements with the same attributes, such as intensity, depth, color and texture. Therefore, the use of segmentation techniques allows us to identify specific anatomical structures. Some brain segmentation methods are able to identify white matter (WM), gray matter (GM) and cerebrospinal fluid structures (CSF), others allow us to isolate and quantify a specific brain anatomical area, such as a multiple sclerosis lesion, a brain tumor or subcortical structures [9].

Brain segmentation suffers from many issues that should be avoided and corrected. The first is the noise of the image—a noisy image does not permit good delineation of the boundaries of brain structures. Another is that the inhomogeneity of intensity, the non-uniformity in the radio frequency (RF) field during data acquisition, results in the shading of the effect. Finally, the partial volume effect occurs when more than one type of class occupies one pixel or voxel of an image [9].

De-noising methods are used to address the issue of noise. To remove noise from an MRI image is difficult, and usually standard or advanced filters are used, such as linear filtering methods, anisotropic nonlinear diffusion filtering, Markov random field statistical analysis, wavelet models and analytically correction methods. Standard linear filters modify the value of a pixel by the average of the neighbor. These filters reduce noise but degrade image details and the edges of the image appear blurred [10]. Advanced filters perform better in terms of preserving the edges of the images.

Intensity inhomogeneity is a smooth spatially varying function that changes the intensity inside originally homogeneous regions. It is independent of noise. Inhomogeneity correction models can be divided into prospective methods and retrospective methods [10–13]. In prospective methods inhomogeneity is corrected by estimating the inhomogeneity field of the MRI acquisition system. Retrospective methods are more general and do not assume any information about the acquisition methods. They can correct both MR scanner-induced and patient induced inhomogeneity [10, 14].

8.9 Image segmentation methods

In *intensity thresholding* a threshold is established and the image is divided into groups of pixels with a value greater or smaller than the established value [9]. This technique is very easy to use and well suited for dividing CSF from brain tissue in T2 weighted images, but is not applicable for structures with a complex mesh of intensity, such as an intracerebral mass. There are different algorithms for different thresholding methods, such as global thresholding, adaptive thresholding, optimal global thresholding and adaptive thresholding [9, 15].

In *region growing* the aim is to find a pixel or a group of pixels of the region that needs to be segmented. These selected image elements are called seeds, and are used as a standard to identify and to choose pixels with the same characteristics. Region growing analysis allows one to identify structures with the same image characteristics. It is also possible to subdivide regions that are not uniform with the area of interest and this procedure is called splitting.

Edge detection techniques are used for evaluating regions that have good contrast and where the exact limits, defined by two different gray scale intensity values, allow the edge detection analysis to identify boundaries between the structure or the tissue of interest and the other structures with different intensity. The disadvantages of these mathematical operators are that they suffer from problems such as over-segmentation, sensitivity to noise, poor detection of significant areas with low contrast boundaries and poor detection of thin structures.

Using *classifiers*, the image is divided into partitions using training data with known labels as references.

Clustering is the process of organizing objects into groups to differentiate structures or clusters present in a collection of unlabeled data. Two types of clustering are K-means clustering and fuzzy c-means clustering, which allows more flexibility by introducing multiple fuzzy membership grades to multiple clusters.

The aim of *statistical models* is to resolve segmentation issues by assigning a class label to a pixel or by estimating the relative amounts of the various tissue types within a pixel. Such models include expectation maximization and Markov random fields.

Artificial neural networks (ANNs) are parallel networks of processing elements or nodes to simulate neural networks, where each node is able to execute a basic computational task. By using training data, spatial classification can be obtained and classified.

Deformable models are techniques for detecting region boundaries by using close parametric curves or surfaces that deform under the influence of internal or external forces. To delineate an object boundary in an image, a closed curve or surface must be placed near the desired boundary and then undergoes an iterative relaxation process. External forces are usually derived from the image to drive the curve or surface toward the desired feature of interest. Deformable models are generally used for cerebral cortical segmentation. They are capable of generating closed parametric curves or surfaces from images and incorporating a smoothness constraint that provides robustness to noise and spurious edges.

The *atlas guided approaches* are methods that use a brain atlas to provide knowledge which can help in grouping the segments into anatomical structures, to obtain a fully automated cortical segmentation procedures. Atlases are created by using different data from different subjects. The first step of this technique is called 'atlas warping' and consists of a transformation that maps a pre-segmented atlas image to the target image, such as a registration based process. Atlas-based segmentation should be used to segment structures that are stable over the population of study. If the contrast of the image is optimal, atlas-based segmentation is the best choice. The disadvantage is that it requires a rigid and complex registration, because the image should be registered to the atlas before segmentation [10].

Brain parenchymal fraction (BPF) is the ratio of the brain parenchymal tissue volume to the total volume within the surface contour of the whole brain. This method uses an algorithm to identify structures other than the brain, such as cranial teca and external CSF spaces, and subtracts them from the brain tissue. The major advantage of this technique is that variations over time in the field of view, scanner gradient strengths and positioning within the scanner do not influence the quantification of brain atrophy. It is reported that automated segmentation using BPF does not always provide satisfactory automatic brain segmentation, while semi-automatic methods suffer from great variability. Moreover, intra-sulcal subarachnoid CSF spaces are not evaluated, and could invalidate a finding of peripheral sovra-tentorial atrophy.

In calculating the *brain to intracranial capacity ratio* (BICCR), the T2 weighted image is normalized for intensity and head size, and a de-noising filter is applied to reduce noise within the image. Then voxels are classified into gray matter, white matter, cerebrospinal fluid and inflammatory lesions, and each volume is calculated. This method suffers from the partial volume effect.

SPM based segmentation uses SPM, software which allows brain tissue segmentation by identifying pixel values and classifying them by the value of intensity into white matter, gray matter and CSF image elements. Before this operation an algorithm is applied to reduce image inhomogeneity and to remove extracranial tissues and then the image, positioned in a stereotactical space, is normalized with a brain atlas. The main issue is that white matter lesions are always included in the brain volume calculation. To avoid this problem it is possible to manually define white matter lesions by calculating the BPF using the sum of GM, WM and lesion volumes divided by the sum of GM, WM, lesion volumes and CSF volumes. Alternatively, the lesion volumes could be subtracted and voxels previously classified as GM and WM are conditionally dilated and then divided by the sum of GM, WM and CSF. The SPM segmentation technique is used to calculate the WM and GM fractions, which are quite useful in the evaluation of multiple sclerosis patient images.

Structural image evaluation using normalization of atrophy-cross-sections (SIENAX) is a fully automated algorithm to estimate volume measurements by using a brain extraction tool to segment the brain tissue from the non-brain tissue and to estimate the outer skull surface. SIENAX can also estimate white and gray matter volumes.

Fuzzy connected principles, based on the theory of fuzzy connectedness, have been applied to segment brains and specifically to quantify multiple sclerosis brain volume losses. This theory uses different signal contrasts to segment the brain from the other structures and white matter from gray matter. Dual-echo fast spin-echo MR sequences are used. An operator indicates a few points in the images by identifying the white matter, the gray matter and the CSF. Each of these objects is then detected as a fuzzy connected set. The holes in the union of these objects correspond to potential lesion sites which are utilized to detect each potential lesion as a 3D fuzzy connected object. These objects are presented to the operator who indicates acceptance/rejection through the click of a mouse button. The number and volume of accepted lesions is then computed and outputted.

In the *seed-growing technique* the operator puts an ROI into the tissue which needs to be segmented. Then this seed grows and the ROI includes every voxel with an intensity included within the highest and lowest threshold values. These values can be automatically or manually defined. Also, boundaries can be manually corrected. The limitations of this technique are that it is relatively time-consuming and does not have good reproducibility, and also suffers somewhat from inter- and intra-observer variability.

The algorithm applied in the *histogram segmentation* technique is able to analyze the histogram of the intensities of T2 and PD images and to automatically establish intensity value thresholds which can be used to separate brain tissues from non-brain tissues. The results mask the T1 weighted images to establish the GM, WM and CSF.

Central cerebral volume is the volume of brain tissue of each 2D slice from the velum interpositum cerebri (which is considered to be stable in brain atrophy) to the skull is calculated and an algorithm automatically extracts the brain from the skull and CSF on selected slices.

CSF measures, using an automated intensity based technique, define the high boundary between CSF and brain tissue for an MR acquisition, define the CSF limits and evaluate ventricular volumes.

8.10 Registration based methods

Registration means overlapping two images to find differences and similarities, and registration based measurement allows us to evaluate the change in volume of two different time point images of the same patient, to obtain the absolute volume [15]. The information that can be obtained by the analysis methods is not only an absolute measure, it also provides regional data about localized atrophy [15]. Additionally, registration based methods allow one to avoid the intrinsic problems of reproducibility of the segmentation based methods, that could hide or underestimate small changes in volume, because of the intrinsically error prone segmentation techniques. The main difficulty for registration based analysis is the need for the images to be spatially matched or, in other terms, to be spatially registered.

Structural imaging evaluation with normalization for atrophy (SIENA) is an automated method that uses a tessellated mesh to model the brain surface. While the brain surface is identified by using a local threshold and a smoothness factor, the outer skull is used to constrain the registration while normalizing the image to geometrical changes.

Segmentation propagation is a technique which registers serial images using an automated rigid body registration algorithm that detects crest-lines in the images and matches points corresponding to a maximum curvature in the principal directions. Intensity scaling is performed so that serial images will have the same average intensity and automated non-rigid registration is used to calculate displacement vectors and compute residual deformation between serial images that are not accounted for by rigid body registration. The residual deformation field is applied to a segmentation of the baseline brain and is automatically propagated through any number of serial images to provide an estimate of volume change.

8.11 Lesion segmentation

As in whole brain volume analysis, we distinguish automated methods and semi-automated methods to quantitatively describe the multiple sclerosis lesion load. Moreover, the algorithms applied for this kind of analysis are based on the same principles, such as image thresholding, intensity gradient features, intensity histogram modeling of the expected tissue classes, identification of the nearest neighbour or fuzzy connectedness [8].

A semi-automated approach seems to be preferable because datasets have differences in tissue contrast and operator intervention is required to verify correct lesion segmentation [8]. Indeed, intra- and inter-observer reproducibility of contouring are better than for manual segmentation but the method is still labor intensive.

8.12 Conclusion

In the last few years several techniques have been proposed for the detection and quantification of brain volume, lesions and degree of atrophy, and we have now reached an excellent level of detail with the advantage that most of the processes that previously required human work are now almost completely automated.

References

[1] Ferguson B, Matyszak M K, Esiri M M and Perry V H 1997 Axonal damage in acute multiple sclerosis lesions *Brain* **120** 393–9

[2] Minagar A, Toledo E G, Alexander J S and Kelley R E 2004 Pathogenesis of brain and spinal cord atrophy in multiple sclerosis *J. Neuroimaging* **14** 5S–10S

[3] Fisher E *et al* 2002 Eight-year follow-up study of brain atrophy in patients with MS *Neurology* **59** 1412–20

[4] Chard D T and Miller D H 2009 What you see depends on how you look: gray matter lesionsin multiple sclerosis *Neurology* **73** 918–9

[5] Chard D and Miller D 2009 Is multiple sclerosis a generalized disease of the central nervous system? An MRI perspective *Curr. Opin. Neurol.* **22** 214–8

[6] Siffrin V, Vogt J, Radbruch H, Nitsch R and Zipp F 2010 Multiple sclerosis—candidate mechanisms underlying CNS atrophy *Trends Neurosci.* **33** 202–10

[7] Haines J D, Inglese M and Casaccia P 2011 Axonal damage in multiple sclerosis *Mt Sinai J. Med.* **78** 231–43

[8] Vrenken H *et al* 2013 MAGNIMS Study Group. Recommendations to improve imaging and analysis of brain lesion load and atrophy in longitudinal studies of multiple sclerosis *J. Neurol.* **260** 2458–71

[9] Xu J and Potenza M N 2012 White matter integrity and five-factor personality measures in healthy adults *Neuroimage.* **59** 800–7

[10] Balafar M A, Ramli A R and Mashohor S 2011 Brain magnetic resonance image segmentation using novel improvement for expectation maximizing *Neurosciences* **16** 242–7

[11] Yang Y, Ruan S and Wu B 2018 Efficient segmentation and correction model for brain MR images with level set framework based on basis functions *Magn. Reson. Imaging* **54** 249–64

[12] Shboul Z A, Reza S M S and Iftekharuddin K M 2018 Quantitative MR image analysis for brain tumor *VipIMAGE 2017* **27** 10–8

[13] Ji Z, Xia Y and Zheng Y 2017 Robust generative asymmetric GMM for brain MR image segmentation *Comput. Methods Programs Biomed.* **151** 123–38

[14] Chang H, Huang W, Wu C, Huang S, Guan C, Sekar S, Bhakoo K K and Duan Y 2017 A new variational method for bias correction and its applications to rodent brain extraction *IEEE Trans. Med. Imaging* **36** 721–33

[15] Miller D H, Barkhof F, Frank J A, Parker G J and Thompson A J 2002 Measurement of atrophy in multiple sclerosis: pathological basis, methodological aspects and clinical relevance *Brain* **125** 1676–95

IOP Publishing

Neurological Disorders and Imaging Physics, Volume 1
Application of multiple sclerosis
Luca Saba and Jasjit S Suri

Chapter 9

MR spectroscopy in multiple sclerosis

Michele Porcu, Paolo Garofalo, Jasjit S Suri and Luca Saba

Proton MR spectroscopy (^{1}H-MRS) is a widely used MR technique that is able to identify and to characterize the chemical composition of both normal and pathological brain tissues. The metabolic spectrum of chronic multiple sclerosis revealed by ^{1}H-MRS is characterized by dynamic changes in the metabolite profile of the lesions according to the phase of disease and the cerebral region analysed. ^{1}H-MRS in MS is mainly used in clinical practice as a supplementary technique for differential diagnosis of tumefactive demyelinating lesions (TDLs) with tumoral lesions.

9.1 Introduction

Proton MR spectroscopy (^{1}H-MRS) is a widely used MR technique that is able to identify and to characterize the chemical composition of both normal and pathological brain tissues [1–4]. Although its use in routine clinical studies of multiple sclerosis (MS) remains limited mainly due to technical disadvantages [2], it can provide several types of useful information for differential diagnosis between MS and other lesions (for example gliomas [5]), and for MS assessment, particularly in research [3].

From a technical point of view, MR spectroscopy is able to record signals from metabolites present in a specific tissue [1]. Metabolites are characterized by specific resonances or peaks in the resonance spectrum as functions of frequency, commonly expressed as the shift in parts-per-million (ppm) relative to a standard [1, 3]. In clinical practice, *in vivo* ^{1}H-MRS analyzes carbon-bound protons in the 1–5 ppm range of the chemical shift scale [3]. We can identify several important peaks in a typical ^{1}H-MRS spectrum: the neural metabolite *N*-acetylaspartate (NAA), the glial metabolite myo-inositol (mIns), choline containing compounds such as glycerophosphocholine and phosphocholine (tCho), neurotransmitters γ-aminobutyric acid (GABA), glutamate (Glu) and glutamine (Gln), other important metabolites such as phosphocreatine and creatine (tCr), lactate (Lac) and macromolecules (MM) [3]. Spectra can be obtained from one selected brain region using the 'single-voxel'

doi:10.1088/2053-2563/ab1fdcch9

technique, or from multiple regions using the 'multivoxel' technique [1, 3]. The shape of the spectrum and the ratio of the metabolites are the parameters that give us the main information on the metabolic content of the region of tissue analysed [1, 3].

The main features of MS lesions revealed by ^{1}H-MRS will be explored in the following sections.

9.2 ^{1}H-MRS in MS: general concepts

Multiple sclerosis is primarily an inflammatory disease of the brain and spinal cord, characterized by focal lymphocytic infiltration and damage to myelin and axons [6]. The aetiology is unknown, and the McDonald diagnostic criteria [7], a combination of clinical, radiographic and laboratory criteria, are commonly used for diagnosis of MS.

MS lesions can be located along the perivenular space in all the central nervous system (CNS) structures in the deep, periventricular or juxtacortical white matter, or at the white matter/grey matter interface. Lesions are typically hyperintense on T2-weighted sequences, fluid attenuated inversion recovery (FLAIR) and double inversion recovery (DIR) sequences, and iso- to hypointense on T1-weighted sequences [8]. Active plaques can appear hyperintense on post-contrast T1-weighted images, and show restricted diffusion on diffusion weighted imaging (DWI) sequences [8].

The metabolic spectrum of chronic multiple sclerosis revealed by ^{1}H-MRS is characterized by dynamic changes in the metabolite profile of the lesions according to the phase of disease (from acute to chronic stages) and the cerebral region analysed, in particular normal-appearing white matter (NAWM), grey matter (GM) and normal-appearing grey matter (NAGM), and following therapy [4, 8, 9].

9.3 Acute MS lesions

It has been demonstrated that acute MS lesions show increased levels of lipids [9, 10], mIns [9, 11], MM [3], tCho and Lac [8, 9, 11], and reduced levels of NAA [8, 9, 12].

Changes in tCho and lipid levels reflect the release of membrane phospholipids, whereas the increased levels of Lac are due to the metabolism of inflammatory cells. Decreased levels of NAA reflect neuroaxonal loss or dysfunction [8, 9]. Elevated tCho/tCr with normal or reduced NAA/tCr is typical [8, 14] (table 9.1).

9.4 Chronic MS lesions

After the acute phase, Lac levels in MS lesions tend to decrease progressively and normalize in a variable period of time (from days to weeks), whereas tCho and lipids tend to return to normal values over several months. On the other hand NAA levels tend to remain reduced or to partially recover soon after the acute phase [8].

Chronic MS lesions are then characterized by low or normal levels of lipids, Lac and Glu, reduced levels of NAA, variable levels of tCho and increased levels of mIns [8–10, 14] (table 9.1).

Table 9.1. Metabolite levels according to the lesion/region of brain analyzed.

	Lesion/region of brain		
Metabolite levels	Acute MS lesion	Chronic MS lesion	NAWM, GM and NAGM
NAA	Elevated	Reduced or partial recovery	Reduced[c]
Lipids	Elevated	Normal or reduced[a]	Elevated
mIns	Elevated	Elevated	Elevated or reduced
MM	Elevated	—	—
tCho	Elevated	Elevated or reduced[b]	Elevated
Lac	Elevated	Normal or reduced[a]	—
tCho/tCr	Elevated	—	Reduced
NAA/tCr	Normal or elevated	Reduced or partial recovery	Reduced
Glu, Gln and GABA	—	—	Elevated

[a] Tend to normalize over several months.
[b] Tend to normalize from days to weeks.
[c] More consistent in GM in the early stages of the disease.
MS = multiple sclerosis; NAWM = normal-appearing white matter; GM = grey matter; NAGM = normal-appearing grey matter; NAA = *N*-acetylaspartate; mIns = myo-inositol; MM = macromolecules; Lac = lactate; tCho = choline containing compounds such as glycerophosphocholine and phosphocholine; tCr = phosphocreatine and creatine; Glu, Gln and GABA = neurotransmitters glutamate, glutamine and γ-aminobutyric acid.

9.5 NAWM, GM and NAGM

Several studies indicate that the NAWM of patients with MS are characterized by low NAA levels compared to healthy controls [8, 9, 15–17], and this fact is commonly attributed to axonal damage, which is more pronounced in advanced disease stages [2]. As well as active MS lesions, NAWM is characterized by increased lipids, mIns [10], tCr [18] and tCho [19]. Further, Glu and GABA levels, which are markers of neurotoxicity, increases [13]. A recent study by Fleischer *et al* [20] performed a metabolic comparison between NAWM and chronic MS lesions using ^{1}H-MRS, finding similar concentrations of multiple metabolites, suggesting that microglia activation is not limited to MS chronic lesions but tends to manifest diffusely across the NAWM.

Similarly to NAWM, grey matter and NAGM show increased levels of lipids and decreased levels of NAA, Glu, GABA and tCho, with variable levels of tCr and mIns [10]. In GM, NAA decreased levels are more consistent in the early stages of disease (table 9.1) [2, 21–23].

9.6 MS therapy

Different studies using ^{1}H-MRS analysed metabolic changes of the brain following therapies with interferon-β (IFN-β), glatiramer acetate, biotin and natalizumab [9].

The influence of IFN-β treatment on NAA levels showed controversial results [24, 25], as well as Cho levels [26, 27].

Table 9.2. Changes in metabolite levels according to the treatment.

Treatment	Effects on metabolites
IFN-β	Decrease or increase of NAA and tCho [24–27]
Glatiramer acetate	Increase of NAA and tCho after treatment [28]
	No differences with placebo [29]
Biotin	Normalization of tCho levels in NAWM [30]
Natalizumab	Increase of NAA and tCr after treatment [31]

NAA = *N*-acetylaspartate; tCho = choline containing compounds such as glycerophosphocholine and phosphocholine; NAWM = normal-appearing white matter; tCr = phosphocreatine and creatine.

Controversial results were also found for glatiramer acetate treatment. In fact, one study [28] evidenced increased levels of NAA after four years of treatment, while another study that compared glatiramer to placebo in patients with primary progressive MS did not find any statistical differences in NAA and tCho levels between the two cohorts [29].

High doses of biotin seem to act as a neuroprotective agent in the brain, and one study [30] showed that this drug tends to normalize tCho levels in the NAWM of patients with MS.

Natalizumab, a recombinant monoclonal antibody, seems to increase NAA and tCr levels when compared to IFN-β and glatiramer, and it was suggested that this result is due to improved axonal metabolism [31]. A potential adverse effect of natalizumab treatment in patients who suffer from relapsing–remitting MS is progressive multifocal leukoencephalopathy (PML), due to the reactivation of the John Cunningham virus (JCV). A recent paper by Schneider *et al* [32] studied the metabolic profile of MS patients who suffered from PML using ^{1}H-MRS, concluding that lipids, tCho/tCr and NAA/tCr are relevant markers in a post-PML setting.

A summary of these data is provided in table 9.2.

9.7 ^{1}H-MRS in MS: clinical practice

Even if the continuous technological improvement in hardware and software solutions is helping researchers to better understand the pathological mechanisms underlying MS, ^{1}H-MRS in clinical practice remains challenging. In fact, although several studies have established its technical feasibility and diagnostic accuracy, only a few studies have demonstrated that ^{1}H-MRS has a broad impact on differential diagnosis, patient treatment and outcome [3, 33].

^{1}H-MRS in MS is mainly used in clinical practice as a supplementary technique for differential diagnosis of tumefactive demyelinating lesions (TDLs) and tumoral lesions. A study by Saindane *et al* [34] analyzed the role of multivoxel ^{1}H-MRS in differential diagnosis between TDLs and high-grade gliomas. They found that NAA/tCr differed significantly between TDLs and high-grade gliomas only in central portions of the lesion and not in other parts, and TDLs typically showed higher NAA/tCr compared to gliomas. The authors concluded that caution is needed in spectroscopy data interpretation. Another study by Malhotra *et al* [35]

Table 9.3. Main differential diagnosis criteria between tumefactive demyelinating lesions (TDLs) and other pathological conditions in MR spectroscopy.

Main differential diagnosis	Spectrum differences
Tumoral lesion	TDLs show elevated NAA/tCr in the central portion of the lesion [34]
	TDLs show Glu and Gln peaks in spectroscopy [35]
ADEM	Recovery of NAA levels [36]

ADEM = acute disseminated encephalomyelitis; NAA = *N*-acetylaspartate; tCr = phosphocreatine and creatine; Glu and Gln = glutamate and glutamine.

demonstrated that TDLs show Glu and Gln in spectroscopy, and also that this element can help in differentiating TDLs from neoplastic lesions (table 9.3).

Another important differential diagnosis to be taken into consideration is that with acute disseminated encephalomyelitis (ADEM), and ADEM shows recovery of tNAA signal as a favourable prognostic sign (table 9.3) [3, 36].

Recent research by Llufriu *et al* [37] tried to identify potential markers of the central nervous system in order to predict brain volume loss and clinical disability in MS, and they found that mIns/NAA in NAWM had consistent predictive power for both neurological disability evolution and brain atrophy.

Finally, technological evolution in hardware and software solutions will help researchers and clinicians in expanding the use of ^{1}H-MRS in MS. The use of a 7 T MR scanner could potentially help in finding biochemical markers of MS with high accuracy and reproducibility, as evidenced for example by Prinsen *et al* [38], who were able to precisely quantify glutathione, GABA and Glu in five patients affected by MS in a single 1 h examination using a 7 T MR scanner.

References

[1] Lin A, Ross B D, Harris K and Wong W 2005 Efficacy of proton magnetic resonance spectroscopy in neurological diagnosis and neurotherapeutic decision making *NeuroRx* **2** 197–214

[2] De Stefano N and Filippi M 2007 MR spectroscopy in multiple sclerosis *J. Neuroimaging* **17** 31S–5S

[3] Oz G *et al* 2014 Clinical proton MR spectroscopy in central nervous system disorders *Radiology* **270** 658–79

[4] Sajja B R, Wolinsky J S and Narayana P A 2009 Proton magnetic resonance spectroscopy in multiple sclerosis *Neuroimaging Clin. N. Am.* **19** 45–58

[5] Ikeguchi R *et al* 2018 Proton magnetic resonance spectroscopy differentiates tumefactive demyelinating lesions from gliomas *Mult. Scler. Relat. Disord.* **26** 77–84

[6] Compston A and Coles A 2008 Multiple sclerosis *Lancet* **372** 1502–17

[7] Thompson A J *et al* 2017 Diagnosis of multiple sclerosis: 2017 revisions of the McDonald criteria *Lancet Neurol.* **17** 162–73

[8] Filippi M and Rocca M A 2011 MR imaging of multiple sclerosis *Radiology* **259** 659–81

[9] Mahajan K R and Ontaneda D 2017 The role of advanced magnetic resonance imaging techniques in multiple sclerosis clinical trials *Neurotherapeutics* **14** 905–23

[10] Rovira A and Alonso J 2013 ^{1}H magnetic resonance spectroscopy in multiple sclerosis and related disorders *Neuroimaging Clin. N. Am.* **23** 459–74

[11] De Stefano N *et al* 1995 Chemical pathology of acute demyelinating lesions and its correlation with disability *Ann. Neurol.* **38** 901–9

[12] Richards T L 1991 Proton MR spectroscopy in multiple sclerosis: value in establishing diagnosis, monitoring progression, and evaluating therapy *AJR Am. J. Roentgenol.* **157** 1073–8

[13] Srinivasan R, Sailasuta N, Hurd R, Nelson S and Pelletier D 2005 Evidence of elevated glutamate in multiple sclerosis using magnetic resonance spectroscopy at 3 T *Brain* **128** 1016–25

[14] Narayana P A, Doyle T J, Lai D and Wolinsky J S Serial proton magnetic resonance spectroscopic imaging, contrast-enhanced magnetic resonance imaging, and quantitative lesion volumetry in multiple sclerosis *Ann. Neurol.* **43** 56–71

[15] Ruiz-Peña J L *et al* 2004 Magnetic resonance spectroscopy of normal appearing white matter in early relapsing–remitting multiple sclerosis: correlations between disability and spectroscopy *BMC Neurol.* **4** 8

[16] Fu L *et al* 1998 Imaging axonal damage of normal-appearing white matter in multiple sclerosis *Brain* **121** 103–13

[17] Sarchielli P *et al* 1999 Absolute quantification of brain metabolites by proton magnetic resonance spectroscopy in normal-appearing white matter of multiple sclerosis patients *Brain* **122** 513–21

[18] Inglese M, Li B S and Rusinek H 2003 Diffusely elevated cerebral choline and creatine in relapsing–remitting multiple sclerosis *Magn. Reson. Med.* **50** 190–5

[19] Tartaglia M C *et al* 2002 Choline is increased in pre-lesional normal appearing white matter in multiple sclerosis *J. Neurol.* **249** 1382–90

[20] Fleischer V *et al* 2016 Metabolic patterns in chronic multiple sclerosis lesions and normal-appearing white matter: intra-individual comparison by using 2D MR spectroscopic imaging *Radiology* **281** 536–43

[21] Wylezinska M *et al* 2003 Thalamic neurodegeneration in relapsing–remitting multiple sclerosis *Neurology* **60** 1949–54

[22] Inglese M *et al* 2004 Three-dimensional proton spectroscopy of deep gray matter nuclei in relapsing–remitting MS *Neurology* **63** 170–2

[23] Geurts J J *et al* 2006 MR spectroscopic evidence for thalamic and hippocampal, but not cortical, damage in multiple sclerosis *Magn. Reson. Med.* **55** 478–83

[24] Narayanan S, De Stefano N and Francis G S 2001 Axonal metabolic recovery in multiple sclerosis patients treated with interferon β-1b *J. Neurol.* **248** 979–86

[25] Parry A *et al* 2003 β-interferon treatment does not always slow the progression of axonal injury in multiple sclerosis *J. Neurol.* **250** 171–8

[26] Yetkin M F, Mirza M and Donmez H 2016 Monitoring interferon β treatment response with magnetic resonance spectroscopy in relapsing–remitting multiple sclerosis *Medicine* **95** e4782

[27] Sarchielli P *et al* 1998 ^{1}H-MRS in patients with multiple sclerosis undergoing treatment with interferon β-1a: results of a preliminary study *J. Neurol. Neurosurg. Psychiatry* **64** 204–12

[28] Khan O *et al* 2017 The relationship between brain MR spectroscopy and disability in multiple sclerosis: 20-year data from the US Glatiramer Acetate Extension Study *J. Neuroimaging* **27** 97–106

[29] Sajja B R *et al* 2008 Longitudinal magnetic resonance spectroscopic imaging of primary progressive multiple sclerosis patients treated with glatiramer acetate: multicenter study *Mult. Scler.* **14** 73–80

[30] Sedel F *et al* 2015 High doses of biotin in chronic progressive multiple sclerosis: a pilot study *Mult. Scler. Relat. Disord.* **4** 159–69

[31] Wiebenga O T *et al* 2015 Enhanced axonal metabolism during early natalizumab treatment in relapsing–remitting multiple sclerosis *AJNR Am. J. Neuroradiol.* **36** 1116–23

[32] Schneider R *et al* 2017 Metabolic profiles by ^{1}H-magnetic resonance spectroscopy in natalizumab-associated post-PML lesions of multiple sclerosis patients who survived progressive multifocal leukoencephalopathy (PML) *PLoS One* **12** e0176415

[33] Lin A P, Tran T T and Ross B D 2006 Impact of evidence-based medicine on magnetic resonance spectroscopy *NMR Biomed.* **19** 476–83

[34] Saindane A M *et al* 2002 Proton MR spectroscopy of tumefactive demyelinating lesions *AJNR Am. J. Neuroradiol.* **23** 1378–86

[35] Malhotra H S *et al* 2009 Characterization of tumefactive demyelinating lesions using MR imaging and *in vivo* proton MR spectroscopy *Mult. Scler.* **15** 193–203

[36] Bizzi A, Uluğ A M, Crawford T O, Passe T, Bugiani M, Bryan R N and Barker P B 2001 Quantitative proton MR spectroscopic imaging in acute disseminated encephalomyelitis *AJNR Am. J. Neuroradiol.* **22** 1125–30

[37] Llufriu S *et al* 2014 Magnetic resonance spectroscopy markers of disease progression in multiple sclerosis *JAMA Neurol.* **71** 840–7

[38] Prinsen H *et al* 2016 Reproducibility measurement of glutathione, GABA, and glutamate: towards *in vivo* neurochemical profiling of multiple sclerosis with MR spectroscopy at 7 T *J. Magn. Reson. Imaging* **45** 187–98

IOP Publishing

Neurological Disorders and Imaging Physics, Volume 1
Application of multiple sclerosis
Luca Saba and Jasjit S Suri

Chapter 10

MR imaging and multiple sclerosis differential diagnosis

Gerardo Dessì, Vincenzo Secchi, Maria Elisabetta Barraccu, Thanis Saksirinukul and Luca Saba

Magnetic resonance (MR) imaging has become an officially accepted tool in the diagnosis and monitoring of multiple sclerosis (MS) due to the ability of MR to represent and depict the pathologic features of this disease in detail.

Acute multiple sclerosis (MS) plaques show destruction and loss of myelin and occur in a perivenular distribution. They are associated with infiltration of mononuclear cells and lymphocytes. The perivascular demyelination gives the appearance of a finger pointing along the axis of the vessel and in the literature these elongated lesions have been named *Dawson's fingers*. This probably reflects the perivascular inflammation along a penetrating medullary vein.

Active demyelination is accompanied by transient breakdown of the blood–brain barrier. Chronic lesions predominantly show gliosis. MS plaques are distributed throughout the white matter of the optic nerves, cerebrum, chiasm and tracts, brainstem, cerebellum and spinal cord [1].

In 2001 MR imaging was formally included in the diagnostic work-up for patients suspected of having MS by an international panel of MS experts under the auspices of the International Federation of MS Societies, chaired by Ian McDonald. The new criteria replaced the older Poser criteria and have become known as the 'McDonald criteria,' after their lead author. The McDonald criteria recognize the high sensitivity of MRI in detecting and depicting lesions. In 2005, a revision to the McDonald criteria was proposed and adopted to clarify the definition of terms such as 'positive MRI', 'attack', 'dissemination', etc. The 2010 revised McDonald criteria refer to the spatial and chronological distribution of MS. Dissemination in space requires at least one white matter hyperintensity (WMH) in at least two typical locations, while dissemination in time requires non-enhancing and contrast-enhancing lesions in a single MR imaging exam or the development of new lesions at follow-up MR imaging [2, 3].

doi:10.1088/2053-2563/ab1fdcch10

MR imaging has superior sensitivity to demonstrate gross tissue pathology in the brain and spinal cord of MS patients, conventionally providing the diagnosis, treatment response and natural history of the disease [4]. The main pathology is multiple white matter lesions, presenting as a hyperintense signal on fluid sensitive sequences such as T2-W images and fluid attenuation inversion recovery (FLAIR) images. The majority of the lesions are located periventricularly, at the centrum semiovale and callososeptal interface. Other frequent sites are subcortical white matter, the corpus callosum, optic nerves, internal capsule, cerebellar peduncles, brainstem and spinal cord. The appearance of demyelinating lesions can be small, large or confluent, some having a hyperintense rim in T1-W images, and lesions usually appear smaller in size in T1-W images than in T2-W images [5]. Atypical lesions and mass-like lesions occur frequently.

Multiple sclerosis plaques are best displayed with FLAIR and T2-WI sequences. T2-WI images are more sensitive in the posterior fossa, while FLAIR is superior in the supratentorial region, particularly for periventricular lesions closely apposed to an ependymal surface. Gadolinium enhanced T1-weighted MR sequences allow one to distinguish active lesions from inactive lesions, considering that enhancement occurs as a result of increased blood–brain barrier permeability and correlates to areas of inflammation. Lesions that consistently appear dark on pre- and post-contrast T1-weighted images (also known as 'black holes') are related to more severe tissue damage (both demyelination and axonal damage).

Although involvement of the gray matter (GM) was described in the earliest pathology studies of MS [6], cortical lesions are difficult to appreciate in conventional MR images [7] because they are usually small, present poor contrast against normal GM, and can be obscured by partial volume effects from the surrounding cerebral fluid. Double inversion recovery (DIR) MR sequences use two inversion times to suppress the signal from both white matter (WM) and cerebrospinal fluid. The use of DIR sequences has significantly improved the ability of MR imaging to represent cortical lesions (they will appear as hyperintense areas). An increase of 538% in sensitivity has been reported with the use of DIR MR imaging in comparison to T2-weighted sequences [8]. In fact, DIR images show very good delineation of intracortical lesions, which may be mistaken for a juxtacortical lesion or a partial volume artifact on the T2-weighted image and may even be missed on the FLAIR image (figures 10.1(a), (b)).

It is worth noting that the DIR sequence suffers from low signal-to-noise ratio (SNR) and is susceptible to flow artifacts. Newer strategies have been proposed to allow reliable detection of GM lesions. These include the use of a sagittal single-slab 3D DIR sequence and its combination with other techniques such as phase-sensitive inversion recovery detection and 3D magnetization-prepared rapid acquisition with a gradient-echo (GRE) sequence [9, 10]. Nevertheless, detecting cortical lesions in MS patients remains a challenge, particularly for subpial lesions.

The 2010 revision of the McDonald criteria permits making a diagnosis of MS on a single MRI study when certain criteria (table 10.1) are found in a patient with typical clinical features [2].

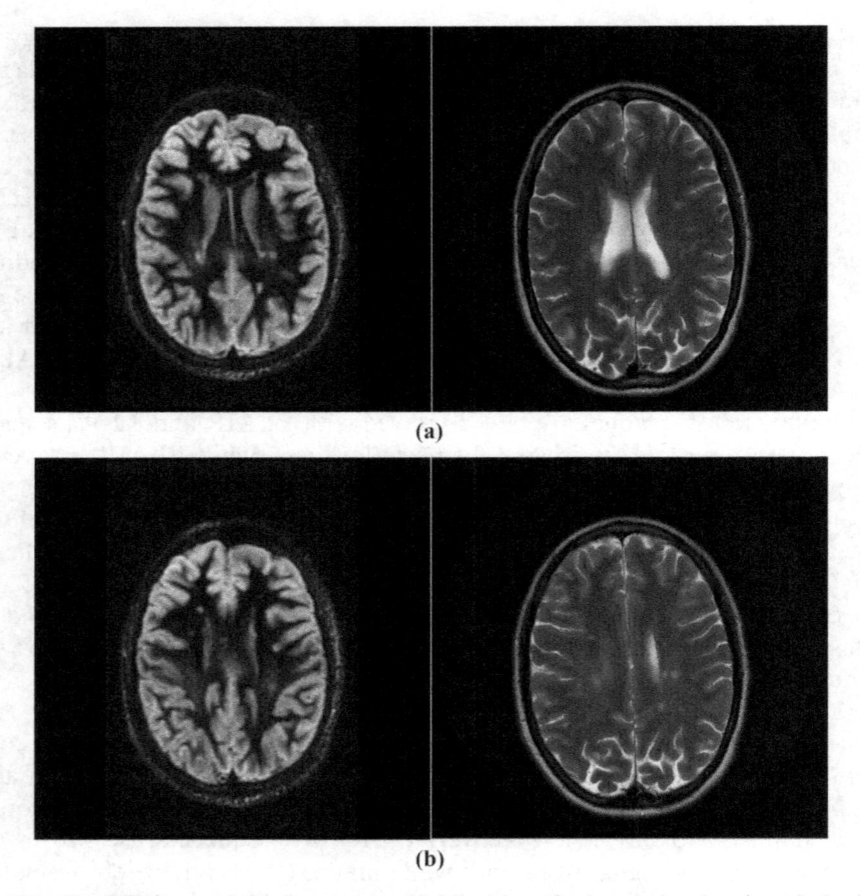

Figure 10.1. The DIR images (left) show very good delineation of subcortical and periventricular lesions, which may be mistaken as partial volume artifacts on the T2-weighted images (right) and may even be missed.

In order to achieve an adequate diagnosis, the following criteria must be met: (1) optimal MRI images are required; (2) a radiologist with a precise understanding of clinical information should make the acquisition; (3) an expert radiologist should be employed to detect typical and atypical findings in the MRI; and (4) to allow differential diagnosis, the radiologist should be aware of other similar pathology patterns in MRI [11].

The new revised criteria suggested by the European Magnetic Resonance Network in Multiple Sclerosis (MAGNIMS) Study Group in 2016, have been launched due to prominent new publications of advanced MRI techniques since 2010 which demonstrate the dissemination of MS lesions in time and space. The new modified criteria are: (1) dissemination in space is documented as an increase of MS lesions in the periventricular white matter from one to three; (2) dissemination in space is also documented as additionally detecting an optic nerve lesion; and (3) for children aged 11 years or older whose clinical context is inconsistent with acute disseminated encephalomyelitis, MS MRI criteria could be applied. The MAGNIMS study group

Table 10.1. Summary of the McDonald criteria for the diagnosis of multiple sclerosis (MS) in a patient with clinically suspected MS.

Demonstration of disease dissemination in space (DIS) requires one or more T2-weighted lesion(s) to be seen in two of the four following areas:

Periventricular	Juxtacortical	Infratentorial	Spinal cord
• Plaques extending along the perivascular veins through the corpus callosum give rise to the relatively specific 'Dawson's fingers' of MS. • White matter abutting the temporal horns and trigones of the lateral ventricles are also highly suggestive.	• Plaques that lie adjacent to, but do not touch, the cortex. • A highly specific site for MS.	• Common regions affected include the floor of the fourth ventricle, cerebellar peduncle and surface of the pons.	• Often in the cervical cord and conus medullaris. • Affects a length of no more than two vertebral segments and <50% of the cross-sectional area. • Usually within the postero-lateral portion of the cord. • An acute cord lesion may expand the cord.

Demonstration of disease dissemination in time (DIT) requires:

1. A new T2-weighted and/or gadolinium-enhancing lesion(s) in follow-up MRI compared to a baseline scan (irrespective of interval duration).
2. The simultaneous presence of asymptomatic gadolinium-enhancing and non-enhancing lesions

Table 10.2. MRI red flags suggestive of an alternative diagnosis to MS. (Modified from the work of The European Magnetic Resonance Network in Multiple Sclerosis group.)

Site affected	'Red flag' MRI feature	Alternative diagnosis
White matter	Normal	ADEM
	Symmetrical distribution of lesions	ADEM
	Absent/rare lesion involving the corpus callosum and periventricular white matter	ADEM
	Absent findings on follow-up MRI after treatment	ADEM, PRES
	Bilateral microhemorrhage	CADASIL, SVD, CAA
	Hemorrhage	PACNS, CAA
	Frequent sparing of corpus callosum and cerebellum	CADASIL, SVD
	T2-weighted-hyperintensity of the temporal lobe, U-fibers at the vertex, external capsule and insular regions	CADASIL
	Simultaneous enhancement of all lesions	PACNS, neurosarcoidosis
	Lesions at the cortical/subcortical junction	PML
	Large lesions with mass effect and enhancement	PACNS
	Multifocal, asymmetrical lesions starting in a juxtacortical location and progressively enlarging	PML
	Punctate enhancement	CLIPPERS, neurosarcoidosis
	Linear or radial pattern of enhancement	PACNS
	Features of restricted diffusion	PML, Susac syndrome, PRES, MTX
Deep gray matter	Lacunar infarcts	SVD, CADASIL
Cortical gray matter	Cortical siderosis	CAA
Spinal cord	Large and swelling lesions	NMO, ADEM
Other	Meningeal enhancement	Susac syndrome, Lyme disease, neurosarcoidosis

Neuromyelitis optica (NMO); acute diffuse encephalomyelitis (ADEM); cerebral autosomal-dominant angiopathy with subcortical infarcts and leukoencephalopathy (CADASIL); small-vessel disease (SVD); progressive multifocal leukoencephalopathy (PML); primary angiitis of the CNS (PACNS); cerebral amyloid angiopathy (CAA): methotrexate (MTX).

have demarcated a series of atypical MRI features, or red flags, which raise suspicion of a different diagnosis (table 10.2).

Peculiarly high levels of iron deposition are frequently found in the brain of MS patients. Potential explanations for the elevated levels of iron in these patients include [12]:

- inflammation, which causes local accumulation of iron due to a disruption of the blood–brain barrier;
- iron-mediated oxidative stress with the development of cytotoxic protein aggregates triggering neurodegeneration;
- amassing of iron-rich macrophages;
- reduced axonal clearance of iron.

This anomalous iron deposition is thought to be the reason for the characteristic hypointensity seen on T2-W images in the dentate nucleus, basal ganglia, thalamus and cortical regions of MS patients. These GM T2 hypointensities have been correlated with the severity of clinical disability and with clinical progression. MR field strength is increasingly sensitive to high iron concentration. With 3.0 T magnets, higher basal ganglia transverse relaxation rates were found in MS patients.

Susceptibility-weighted MR imaging (SWI) has also been used to assess iron concentration and to evaluate cerebral venous oxygenation changes in MS patients.

Table 10.3. Classification of white matter diseases.

Primary demyelinating disease	**Metabolic**
Multiple sclerosis	Osmotic demyelination or central pontine myelinolysis
Baló disease	
Devic disease	
Schilder disease	**Toxic**
Marburg disease	Alcohol
	Radiation
Secondary demyelinating disease	Marchiafava–Bignami disease
Allergic (immunologic)	Disseminated necrotizing leukoencephalopathy
Acute disseminated encephalomyelitis (ADEM)	Drugs, including chemotherapeutic agents and intravenously drugs (cocaine, heroin)
	Toxins (lead, mercury)
Viral	**Dysmyelinating disease**
HIV-associated encephalitis	Alexander disease
Progressive multifocal leukoencephalopathy	Krabbe disease
Subacute sclerosing panencephalitis (SSPE)	Sudanophilic leukodystrophy
	Pelizaeus–Merzbacher disease
Vascular (hypoxic/ischemic)	Canavan disease
Binswanger disease	Metachromatic leukodystrophy
	Adrenoleukodystrophy
CADASIL	
Postanoxic encephalopathy	
Reversible posterior leukoencephalopathy	

SWI sequences demonstrated an increased iron concentration in the deep GM nuclei in MS patients, relative to that in healthy control subjects [13].

Recently, it has been hypothesized that increased iron levels in MS brains are related to anomalies in venous outflow, called chronic cerebrospinal venous insufficiency. Some studies using SWI imaging confirmed a reduced presence of the venous vasculature in the periventricular WM of MS patients, interpreted as a result of decreased oxygen extraction in the affected tissue.

A diagnosis of MS should not only be made on the basis of MRI findings, but should consider the patient's history, clinical signs and symptoms, and adequate laboratory tests. Thanks to improved MRI techniques, it is quite easy to rule out some MS mimickers such as tumors or vascular malformations. However, it remains difficult to differentiate MS lesions from other diseases involving white matter such as Sjögren, neurosarcoidosis, vasculitis (e.g. systemic lupus erythematosus, Behçet disease, …), Lyme disease, acute disseminated encephalomyelitis (ADEM), etc. These disorders may present clinical and MRI findings that are remarkably similar to MS.

In MRI studies, over-diagnosis of MS should be avoided and the radiologist should be aware of potential pitfalls and differential diagnoses. A summary of multifocal white matter lesions is provided in table 10.3.

All these demyelinating syndromes have a common inflammatory factor that injures and sometimes destroys white matter.

Table 10.4. Demyelinating diseases categorized by presumed etiology.

Autoimmune (idiopathic)	**Metabolic/nutritional**
Multiple sclerosis	Osmotic demyelination
Monophasic demyelination	Monophasic Bignami disease
ADEM	Combined systems disease (vitamin B12 deficiency)
Acute hemorrhagic leukoencephalitis	
Optic neuritis (may be the first presentation of MS)	**Toxic**
Acute transverse myelitis (may be the first presentation of MS)	Radiation
	Toxins
	Drugs
Viral	Disseminated necrotizing leukoencephalopathy
Progressive multifocal leukoencephalopathy	
SSPE	
HIV-associated encephalitis	**Trauma**
	Diffuse axonal injury
Vascular (hypoxic/ischemic)	
CADASIL	
Postanoxic encephalopathy	
Reversible posterior leukoencephalopathy	
Binswanger disease	

The oligodendrocyte is the cell responsible for wrapping the axon to build the myelin sheath, and although we speak of white matter diseases as those that affect myelin, in actual fact myelin is not the only brain tissue damaged in 'demyelinating diseases'—axons and neurons are also commonly affected [14]. Our knowledge of these disorders has dramatically improved with more precise histopathology and new MR techniques. We can further divide these diseases based on their presumed etiology (table 10.4).

The location of the involvement of the corpus callosum can also be used to determine some differential diagnosis features between other primary or secondary demyelinating processes (NMO, ADEM, CADASIL, Susac syndrome, PML, Marchiafava–Bignami disease), neoplasms (lymphoma, glioma, gliomatosis cerebri—the latter may mimic white matter disease only by its extension) and traumatic injury (traumatic/DAI-diffuse axonal injury) (table 10.5).

Table 10.5. Corpus callosum involvement: differentiating features of more common causes.

Disease	Location	Imaging characteristics
MS	More frequently the genu and body of the callosum Origin at the callososeptal interface	Small separate lesions ('dot–dash') initially Enhanced in the acute phase
NMO	More frequently the splenium Entire thickness	Larger, overlapping ('marbled') Enhanced in the acute phase
ADEM	Origin at periventricular white matter when present, not from the callososeptal interface	Larger Enhanced in the acute phase; all the lesions may be enhanced at the same time (monophasic)
CADASIL	Entire thickness or central	Usually not enhanced
PML	More frequently the genu and splenium	Usually not enhanced
Susac syndrome	Entire thickness or central	Enhanced in the acute–subacute phase; inflammation and microinfarcts
Marchiafava–Bignami disease	Middle layers of the genu and splenium	Diffusion restriction in the acute phase, atrophy in the chronic phase
Glioma	More frequently the genu and splenium	Enlarged, heterogeneous enhancement, necrosis
Lymphoma	Middle layers of the genu and splenium	Diffusion restriction in the acute phase, atrophy in the chronic phase
Traumatic/diffuse axonal injury	Splenium > genu, grade II disease	Blooming on T2[a]-weighted images Diffusion restriction in acute phase

[a] Cerebral autosomal-dominant arteriopathy with subcortical infarcts and leukoencephalopathy (CADASIL); progressive multifocal leukoencephalopathy (PML).

10.1 Neuromyelitis optica (NMO)

10.1.1 Definition

Neuromyelitis optica, also called Devic's disease, has historically been used for patients with optic neuritis and extensive transverse myelitis.

10.1.2 Pathogenesis

Neuromyelitis optica spectrum disorders are now recognized as being distinct from multiple sclerosis following the identification of aquaporin-4 antibody (AQP4; also termed NMO-IgG). The aquaporin-4 channel is found in astrocytes, and belongs to the family of proteins that conduct water through the cell membrane, and has higher expression along the pathway between the third and fourth ventricles. The antibodies seem to target the regions where the blood–brain barrier is weaker and the expression of aquaporin-4 is higher.

10.1.3 Epidemiology

The prevalence ranges from 0.5 to 4.4 per 100 000 inhabitants, being more common in Asian (overall Indian), and African populations. The age of onset varies, with an average age of 41 years in the USA, about 5–10 years later than typical MS. Women are more commonly affected, with a ratio of 6.5:1. The strong overrepresentation in females suggests that sex hormones play a more significant role than in other autoimmune diseases.

10.1.4 Clinical features

The hallmark clinical features of NMO spectrum disorders are optic neuritis, which is often bilateral or sequential, and longitudinal transverse myelitis, that typically affects three or more vertebral segments with patchy cord and possible thin ependymal enhancement [15]. Patients generally present with subacute visual loss and paraparesis or quadriparesis that might happen simultaneously or in separate successive episodes. Involvement of the brainstem and cervical cord seldom results in life-threatening respiratory compromise. Patients may also have unremitting episodes of nausea, vomiting, or hiccups, usually due to involvement of the brainstem (medulla).

The clinical course of NMO is dominated by relapses that vary in frequency from several per year to attacks separated by many years. In fact, 90% of cases have a recurrent course with more dramatic relapses than MS. If misdiagnosed and treated as ordinary MS, a further exacerbation can be produced. The classic triad of NMO consists of myelitis, optic neuritis (unilateral or bilateral) and positive NMO-immunoglobulins (these have more than 90% specificity and 80% sensitivity for the disease).

10.1.5 Locations and MR appearance

The initial brain MRI in NMO may be normal or demonstrate nonspecific brain white matter lesions that do not fulfil the dissemination in space criteria for MS. MRI obtained in a later phase of NMO can demonstrate lesions in regions of high AQP4 antibody expression. See figures 10.2(a)–(d).

Lesions most often occur in the diencephalon around the third ventricle, around the cerebral aqueduct, and in the anterior midbrain, thalamus and hypothalamus, and are also frequently found in the dorsal brainstem, including the area postrema (dorsal medulla oblongata, described as specific for NMO) and nucleus tractus solitarius, where lesions might be contiguous with those in the cervical spinal cord. Lesions might also be observed in the corpus callosum, but in contrast to MS lesions, in NMO they extend along the long axis of the corpus callosum rather than presenting Dawson's finger appearance.

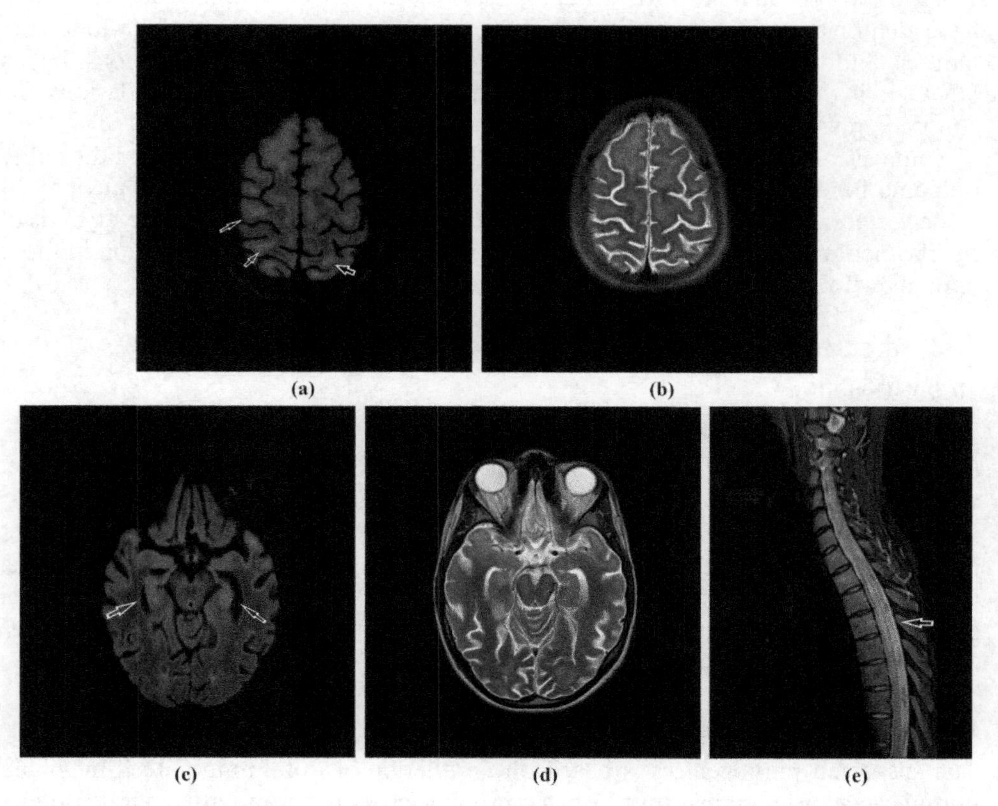

Figure 10.2. Neuromyelitis optica in a 21-year-old woman. (a) Axial FLAIR and (b) T2 images show patchy areas of increased signal involving the frontal and parietal subcortical bilateral regions (arrows in (a)). (c) Axial FLAIR and (d) T2 images show patchy hyperintensities involving the hippocampus bilaterally (arrows in (c)). (e) The sagittal T2-weighted image shows patchy hyperintensity involving the dorsal cord (arrow), consistent with myelitis.

Corpus callosum lesions in NMO preferentially involve the splenium. Compared to those in MS, they are larger, more confluent, more edematous and more heterogeneous. The 'marbled pattern' represents multiple overlapping heterogeneous lesions in the corpus callosum and has been described in the acute phase of NMO. Longitudinally extensive lesions involving the corticospinal tracts can reach the cerebral peduncle and brainstem.

Unlike in MS, myelitis in NMO is longitudinally and transversally extensive, often involving three or more vertebral segments, and is more frequently inhomogeneous. 'Bright spotty lesions' is a newly described spinal finding in NMO, referring to this heterogeneous appearance on axial T2-weighted images and can help differentiate NMO from MS [16].

MRI lesions in deep white matter in patients with NMO can be tumefactive or take the form of nonspecific punctate T2 hyperintensities. Recent studies have described tiny WMHs in the subcortical white matter, usually not traversed by a central venule, in ultra-high magnetic field imaging (7 T) [17].

Furthermore, advanced MR imaging techniques such as diffusion tensor imaging have demonstrated abnormalities in otherwise normal-appearing white and gray matter. Gadolinium enhancement is variable in any of these types of lesions, but in NMO it is generally less discrete than in MS lesions, and in NMO lesions the contrast enhancement might have a cloud-like appearance.

Some lesions resolve completely, which is associated with an improved disability outcome for the patient, but T2 hyperintensity can persist. Focal cord atrophy of some vertebral segments can develop. Longitudinally extensive transverse myelitis of the thoracolumbar cord extending to the conus medullaris is more common in those patients who are seropositive for MOG-IgG.

10.2 Acute disseminated encephalomyelitis (ADEM)

10.2.1 Definition

ADEM is mediated by antigen–antibody complexes and usually occurs in children (typically <15 years old), often within 2 weeks after an antigenic challenge—either a vaccination or an infection (50%–75%, frequently upper respiratory).

ADEM has been identified frequently with antecedent measles, varicella, mumps and rubella infection/vaccination, but is not limited to these infections. Cytomegalovirus (CMV), Epstein–Barr virus (EBV), mycoplasma pneumoniae, myxoviruses, herpes group and HIV infections are also common precipitants. Some cases are absolutely idiopathic.

10.2.2 Pathogenesis

The suspected pathogenesis is based on an allergic or autoimmune (cell-mediated immune response against myelin basic protein) cross-reaction with a viral protein. The pathology of ADEM is characterized by copious perivenular sleeves of demyelination accompanied by an inflammatory infiltrate with huge numbers of macrophages and fewer T and B cells, without the confluent macrophage infiltration and demyelination seen in MS [18].

Detected lesions seem to be of the same pathological stage, unlike in MS, and there is relative axonal sparing. The presence of intracortical microglial collections, particularly in cortical layer three, is a pathognomonic finding in ADEM, which might be the substrate for encephalopathy. These aggregates are accompanied by diffuse meningeal phlogosis, subpial microglial activation and demyelination.

The course is monophasic in 90% of cases, but there is the risk of relapse within the first 12 weeks. Anti-MOG (myelin oligodendrocyte glycoprotein) immunoglobulin G antibodies are present in half of patients with ADEM, and CSF (cerebrospinal fluid) pleocytosis is recurrently present.

The outcome of ADEM is variable. Most patients experience complete recovery, with remarkable improvement or even complete remission at follow-up, although mortality in the initial phase is possible. In fact, although very rare, at the fulminant end of the spectrum of ADEM is acute hemorrhagic leukoencephalitis (Hurst disease) accompanied by diffuse multifocal perivascular demyelination and bleeding confined to the cerebral WM with sparing of the subcortical U-fibers. Hurst disease develops between 1 and 2 weeks after pneumonia and progresses quickly from confusion to coma. Death occurs an average of 1 week after the presentation of symptoms, developing cerebral edema and acute herniation. Histopathologically there is a necrotizing angiitis with petechiae and perivascular hemorrhages.

It is also believed that a subset of patients will later progress to MS, although this could also mean that the first presentation of MS was initially misdiagnosed as ADEM.

10.2.3 Epidemiology

ADEM more commonly affects children and, in contrast to multiple sclerosis, has no sex predilection. It very rarely occurs in adults. The estimated incidence is 0.5–0.8 per 100 000 people per year. In 50%–75% of cases, the clinical onset of disease is preceded by viral or bacterial infections, as previously explained. Although ADEM is quite a rare disease, it is becoming increasingly frequent, because vaccination schedules have expanded over the past few years. Typically, there is a latency of 7–14 days between a febrile illness and the onset of neurologic symptoms. In the case of vaccination-associated ADEM, this latency period may be longer. Incidence is highest in winter and spring, possibly reflecting increased rates of infection.

10.2.4 Clinical features

Patients commonly present with nonspecific symptoms, including headaches, sickness, drowsiness, fever and lethargy. All of these symptoms are quite rare in multiple sclerosis. The course is usually monophasic, although recurrent and multiphasic forms are possible. In general the disease is self-limiting. Neurologic symptoms usually develop subacutely and lead to hospitalization within a week. Some symptoms appear to be age related. In children, long-lasting fever and headaches occur more frequently, while in adults motor and sensory deficits predominate.

According to the International Paediatric MS Study Group, monophasic ADEM is defined as a multifocal clinical syndrome in patients with no history of a prior demyelinating event, including encephalopathic symptoms such as behavioral changes (e.g. irritability, lethargy) or altered consciousness (somnolence). Recurrent ADEM requires another ADEM attack more than 3 months after the first event (after conclusion of corticosteroid therapy), involving the same anatomical area. Multiphasic ADEM requires a second ADEM attack with new areas of involvement.

Sometimes an ADEM attack is the first indicator of the classic relapsing form of MS. In fact, 30% of patients who encounter the ADEM criteria at initial presentation ultimately receive a diagnosis of multiple sclerosis. For this reason, a presumptive diagnosis of ADEM mandates strict clinical and MRI follow-up.

10.2.5 Locations and MR appearance

Unlike lesions in MS, the lesions of ADEM are often large, patchy and poorly marginated in MRI. See figures 10.3(a)–(c). Typically, lesions are located in the subcortical and central WM and cortical gray–white junction of both cerebral hemispheres, the cerebellum, brainstem, optic nerves and spinal cord. The GM of the thalami and basal ganglia is often involved, typically symmetrically. Although variable in size, lesions are commonly larger than 1 cm and present poorly defined margins. Simultaneous enhancement of all lesions is quite infrequent and, although this sign might suggest ADEM, other conditions, such as sarcoidosis or neoplasms, must also be considered. Tumefactive demyelinating lesions can occur in ADEM, but an important differential diagnosis of multiple simultaneously enhancing tumefactive lesions is multifocal primary CNS lymphoma.

Lesions confined to the periventricular WM and corpus callosum are less frequent than in MS. In fact, ADEM is often associated with sparing of the periventricular WM, and thalamic and basal ganglia involvement is seen more frequently than in MS, whereas the latter is suggested by the presence of T1 hypointense 'black holes'.

Four patterns of cerebral involvement have been described based on MRI findings in ADEM [19]: (1) ADEM with small lesions (<5 mm); (2) ADEM with extensive, confluent, or tumefactive lesions and frequent vast perilesional edema and

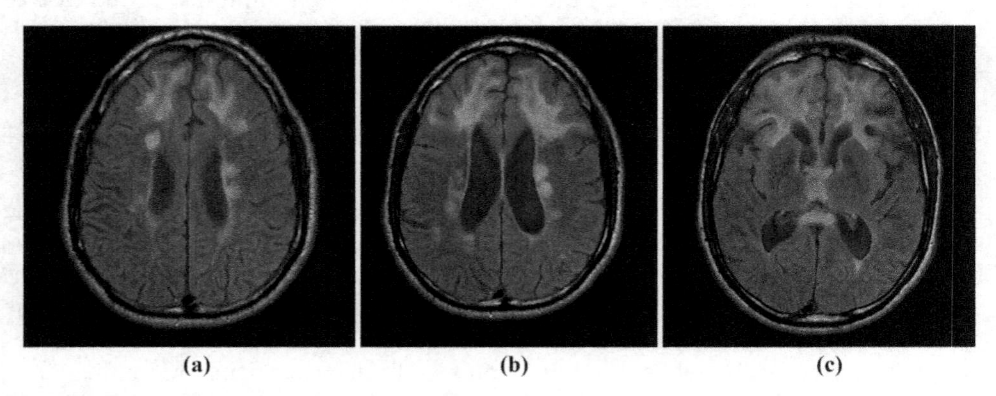

Figure 10.3. Axial FLAIR images of ADEM show some extended areas of hyperintensities located in periventricular white matter, in particular located around the anterior ventricular horn, bilaterally.

mass effects; (3) ADEM with additional symmetric deep GM involvement; and (4) acute hemorrhagic encephalomyelitis.

Lesions in 30%–100% of affected patients show Gd contrast enhancing. The pattern of enhancement is variable: complete or incomplete ring-shaped, nodular, gyral or spotty.

Only about 30% of patients present spinal involvement, predominantly in the thoracic region. The cord lesion is typically large, causing swelling of the cord, and presents variable enhancement. Spinal cord lesions are in fact extensive in ADEM and are usually accompanied by large, poorly defined subcortical WM lesions in brain MRI. In MS patients, in contrast, cord lesions are usually small and commonly associated with subclinical white matter brain lesions of the type seen in MS.

As this pathology is usually monophasic, lesions would be expected to appear simultaneously with the same appearance on contrast-enhanced MRI and are expected to resolve or remain unchanged, with no new lesions in follow-up MR images. Sometimes, however, new lesions are seen in follow-up MRI within the first 3–4 weeks after the initial attack. This fact explains the mixed pattern of enhancing and non-enhancing lesions at the same time point. In some cases there could be a delay of more than 4–6 weeks between the onset of symptoms and the appearance of lesions on MRI and for this reason an initial normal brain MR examination does not exclude this diagnosis.

10.3 Baló's concentric sclerosis

10.3.1 Definition

Baló's concentric sclerosis is a term applied to individual or multiple lesions in the CNS with alternating rings of demyelination and relatively preserved myelin. This sporadic and severe acute monophasic disease is characterized by concentric rims of myelin destruction and repair, showing alternating layers of demyelinated, remyelinated and normal myelinated. The involvement of the centrum semiovale and corona radiata is frequent.

As with tumefactive demyelination, Baló's sclerosis lesions are often mistaken for primary brain tumors and patients frequently undergo biopsy. Although multiple lesions might occur simultaneously, relapse is extremely sporadic. Caution must be taken in interpreting the data for this disease as these generally result from individual cases and small case series.

10.3.2 Pathogenesis

The pathophysiology concerning Baló's concentric sclerosis lesions has long been debated. The most acceptable hypothesis is that lesions arise from a central venule, from which inflammatory mediators spread radially in sequential waves, triggering macrophage-mediated demyelination [20].

One possible explanation for the concentric alternating bands may be that the tissue injury is induced at the edge of the expanding lesion, which induces the expression of neuroprotective proteins to protect the rim of periplaque tissue from damage, thereby resulting in alternate layers of preserved and non-preserved myelinated tissue.

According to the ischemic preconditioning hypothesis, hypoxia-inducible factors are expressed at the leading edge of each successive wave and confer some degree of neuronal and myelin protection, which leads to a concentric appearance. Upregulated expression of hypoxia-inducible proteins, such as HSP70, HIF1A and D110, at lesion borders support this hypothesis.

Other theories suggest lesion growth from a central origin, which is supported by the centrifugal pattern of evolution of lesions on MRI.

10.3.3 Epidemiology

The disorder is very rare, affecting more women than men. It is more common among people of Han Chinese and Filipino descent, in whom MS is less common than among white people.

10.3.4 Clinical features

Patients present with focal neurological signs, or with other symptoms of a cerebral mass, including headache, impaired consciousness, cognitive dysfunction and seizures. Prodromal fever and headache can be associated.

The disease can lead to death in weeks to months. In fact, historically, Baló's concentric sclerosis was considered to have a poor prognosis but now MRI-based assessment has better elucidated the clinical range of lesions, and many patients are now known to recover fully.

10.3.5 Locations and MR appearance

On MRI with T2-W and FLAIR sequences, the lesions appear as concentric rings or whorls with alternating high and low intensity. See figures 10.4(a)–(g). These alternating bands typically show concentric hyperintense bands corresponding to areas of demyelination and gliosis alternating with isointense bands corresponding to normal myelinated white matter.

This pattern can appear as multiple concentric layers (a pathognomonic 'onion-skin lesion': hyperintense–isointense–hypointense concentric rings), as a mosaic, or as a 'floral' configuration. The center of the lesion usually shows no layering because of massive demyelination. In T1-W images alternating bands of hypointensity and isointensity with minimal surrounding edema can be seen. Diffusion-weighted imaging (DWI) often shows peripheral restriction, and Gd enhancement is frequently apparent at the lesion edge, but can also occur in concentric layers.

Other lesions typical of MS are seen simultaneously in up to 55% of patients at presentation. Peripheral restricted diffusion and contrast enhancement often represent the advancing front of demyelination. Simultaneous Baló's sclerosis and tumefactive demyelination has been recently reported in one patient [21] and distinct lesions with mixed radiological and pathological features have been reported, suggesting overlapping mechanisms. Even though Baló's sclerosis was originally described as an acute, monophasic and quickly fatal infection (resembling Marburg

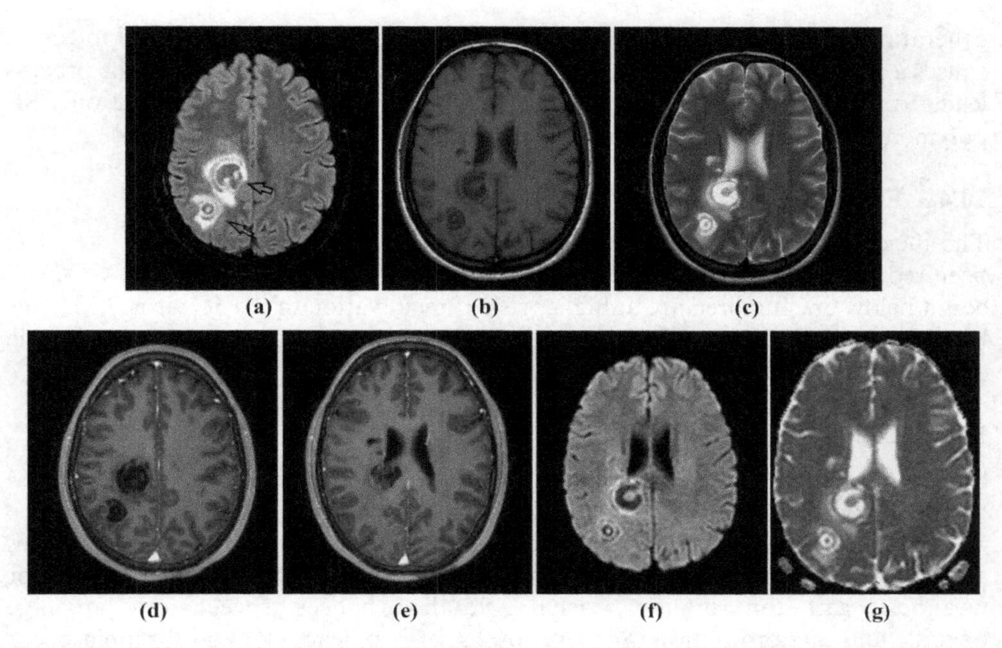

Figure 10.4. Baló concentric sclerosis in a 22-year-old woman. (a) The axial FLAIR image shows extensive simultaneous lamellated white matter lesions in the right parietal lobe (arrows), with involvement of the subcortical U-fibers. Transverse T1-W (b) and T2-W (c) MR images show a striking lamellated pattern of alternating bands of demyelination and relatively normal white matter, reflecting either spared or remyelinated regions. (d) Open-ring gadolinium enhancement on T1-weighted MRI ((e) represents a larger lesion at another level). (f) and (g) The lesions are associated with peripheral restricted diffusion on diffusion-weighted imaging ((f) B1000, (g) ADC map).

disease), large Baló-like lesions are often identified on MRI in patients with a classic acute or chronic MS disease course or in ADEM with a nonfatal course.

10.4 Progressive multifocal leukoencephalopathy (PML)

10.4.1 Definition

PML is a demyelinating disease secondary to reactivation of John Cunningham (JC) virus in immunocompromised patients, such as those suffering from HIV infection/ AIDS (acquired immunodeficiency syndrome) or lymphoproliferative diseases, or transplant patients. The JC virus is a polyomavirus (family Polyomaviridae). This is a ubiquitous virus, asymptomatic infection being present in the normal population and latent persistence in the kidney and cerebrum. Non-AIDS PML linked to immunosuppressive drugs, for example, the monoclonal antibody natalizumab used in MS, is increasingly reported.

10.4.2 Pathogenesis

In patients with PML, JC virus exists in circulating B lymphocytes and is the main characteristic for infection and lysis of oligodendrocytes, which leads to failure in generating myelin and large geographic areas of demyelination. This viral infection causes a progressive destruction of oligodendrocytes, which at the end of the process leads to extensive demyelination. Diagnosis of PML can be made based on CSF polymerase chain reaction analysis for JC viral DNA.

10.4.3 Epidemiology

The incidence of acquired immunodeficiency syndrome (AIDS)-related PML has been reduced with the advent of antiretroviral medication. Patients with a CD4 cell count below one hundred are at higher risk of reactivation of the JC virus. PML has been found in 5%–10% of autopsies in HIV. The diagnosis is supported by the presence of JC antigens in CSF.

10.4.4 Clinical features

Survival was historically poor at 2–6 months, but has improved with antiretroviral therapy, now up to 3–4 years. As any area of the brain may be involved, the clinical appearance is quite varied. Behavioral and cognitive abnormalities are seen in 30%–40% of affected people. Common clinical findings are motor weakness, gait abnormalities, visual field disturbances, speech and language deficits, and incoordination. Sensory loss, seizures, headache and diplopia occur less frequently. Note that PML involves optic radiation resulting in visual deficits, although there is no published optic nerve involvement [22].

10.4.5 Locations and MR appearance

PML lesions present low T1-W, high T2-W and fluid-attenuated inversion recovery (FLAIR) signal in single or multiple rounded to ovoid lesions located on the subcortical U-fibers of WM. See figures 10.5(a)–(g). These are tightly delineated from the overlying cortical GM and are typically asymmetrically distributed and gradually become confluent.

The frontal and parieto-occipital WM, corpus callosum and posterior fossa WM are generally involved. Deep GM impact is less common. In contrast to multiple sclerosis lesions, the periventricular WM is usually spared and spinal cord and Dawson's finger lesions are usually absent. Unlike MS, PML lesions in fact usually occur at the gray–white junction, are frequently monofocal (typically involving the frontal lobes), and may be large, whereas MS lesions are generally located in periventricular areas and are smaller. On T2-W imaging, the affected lesions of PML often have a 'ground glass' appearance. Although very sporadic, crescent shaped high T2-W lesions of the middle cerebellar peduncle have been found in PML patients.

DWI is a crucial sequence in MR imaging in PML as it is not uncommon for acute or subacute PML lesions to show restricted diffusion, a characteristic pattern being a core of facilitated diffusion with a peripheral rim of restricted diffusion [23]. This peculiar look is highly useful when trying to differentiate from MS.

Gd contrast enhancement is habitually lacking due to a relative scarcity of perivascular flogosis, but a subgroup of HIV-positive patients has shown weak

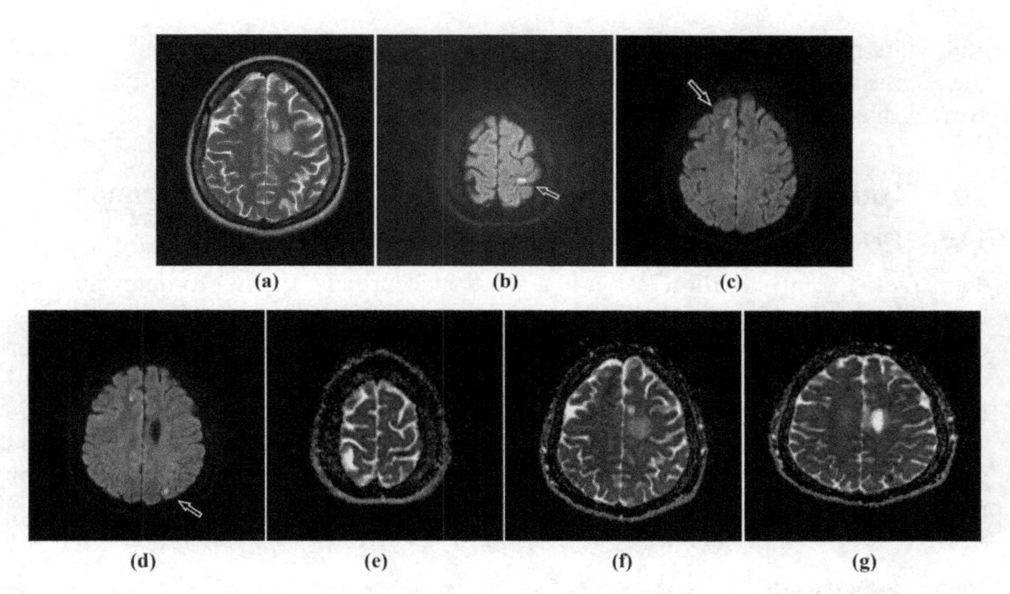

Figure 10.5. PML. A 37-year-old woman affected by MS in follow-up with worsening clinical status. (a) An axial T2 image shows the appearance of a large lesion with edema and blurred borders in the white matter of the left centrum semiovale. (b)–(d) A DWI B1000 series shows the appearance of three small cortical-subcortical frontal and parietal lesions (arrows; two on the left and one on the right hemisphere), with a strong hypersignal and blurred borders. (e)–(g) ADC maps on the same levels as the B1000 series shows the hypointense signal of the lesions, confirming the restricted signal.

peripheral perilesional enhancement. This is a clue differing from the homogeneous or open-ring enhancement usually seen in multiple sclerosis patients. Contrast enhancement can be seen in cases with subsequent immune reconstitution inflammatory syndrome (IRIS) after the beginning of antiretroviral therapy for HIV, in PML related to MS-specific therapy (e.g. natalizumab).

Recent studies have demonstrated that natalizumab-associated PML identified on MRI before the beginning of symptoms is linked to better prognosis. The PML lesions in this subgroup of patients are often located in the frontal lobe subcortical and juxtacortical WM. Brain atrophy is a hallmark of the syndrome.

HIV encephalopathy shares some characteristics with PML: both produce confluent white matter lesions without significant mass effects or contrast enhancing, but these are more peripheral and asymmetric in PML (infecting oligodendrocytes) versus more central and symmetric in HIV encephalopathy (infecting microglia). Distinctions between HIV encephalopathy and PML include a greater tendency for the latter to present subcortical WM hypointensity on T1-weighted imaging and occasional contrast enhancing.

Cytomegalovirus lesions are typically located in the periventricular WM and centrum semiovale. Subependymal contrast enhancing is occasionally observed in cytomegalovirus infected patients.

Other HIV-associated disorders that show hyperintense signal lesions of the WM similar to PML include varicella-zoster leukoencephalitis, ADEM, CNS vasculitis and white matter edema associated with primary or metastatic brain tumors. In all these cases clinical features, laboratory tests and associated MR features allow the correct diagnosis.

10.5 Tumefactive demyelinating lesions (TDL) or pseudotumor

10.5.1 Definition

Tumefactive demyelination lesion is a word inaccurately applied to demyelinating lesions larger than 2 cm in the maximum diameter. This affliction is characterized by cerebral mass lesions, and the symptoms and signs are very similar to those of other demyelinating diseases. Single lesions might be mistaken for neoplasms in MRI and for this reason in the literature the disease also has the name of 'pseudotumour'. TDL can be diagnosed promptly in patients with established MS, although superimposed afflictions mimicking TDLs, such as cerebral abscesses, ischemia or infections, must be considered.

10.5.2 Pathogenesis

The pathogenic process that leads to the development of TDL is very similar to the pathogenic process of MS. It is largely accepted that the development of the inflammatory plaque develops from a breach in the integrity of the blood–brain barrier (BBB) by the interaction of integrins expressed on the shell of lymphocytes.

Genetic and environmental elements, such as viral infections, may facilitate the access of potentially pathogenic autoreactive T cells and antibodies into the CNS via BBB disruption. Inflammatory cytokines within the CNS activate local macrophages, which contribute to tissue injury and demyelination.

TDLs have very high cellularity that may lead to misdiagnosis as glioblastoma, and Creutzfeldt cells may be misinterpreted as mitotic figures. The manifestation of extensive macrophage infiltration is suggestive of demyelination rather than malignant disease. The pathology of TDLs is very similar to that of typical MS lesions with confluent areas of demyelination and relative axonal sparing, even though widespread axonal damage might be observed in TDLs. Additionally, inflammatory aggregates of foamy macrophages are admixed with reactive astrocytes, and perivascular and parenchymal lymphocytic infiltrates are common.

10.5.3 Epidemiology

TDLs have a very similar epidemiology to classic MS. However, it might also occur in people with ADEM or AQP4-IgG-seropositive or MOG-IgG-seropositive NMO spectrum disorders. For this reason, the term tumefactive demyelination is preferred to tumefactive multiple sclerosis. According to some authors, TDL should not be considered as a distinct demyelinating disease, but rather refers to various lesion types encountered in the context of other demyelinating disease processes.

10.5.4 Clinical features

Clinical symptom onset includes seizures, impaired consciousness, cognitive deficits and focal neurological signs. Other symptoms and signs resemble the clinical setting of MS patients. Patients presenting with isolated, diagnostically undifferentiated TDLs seem, in the most recent studies [24], to have better long-term prognosis than patients with conventional multiple sclerosis, but data are still limited.

Slightly elevated concentrations of CSF protein are common findings in patients with TDLs. Patients presenting with a TDL as the first clinical event have CSF-restricted oligoclonal bands less commonly than those in whom lesions grow during the course of proven MS (52% versus 90%).

10.5.5 Locations and MR appearance

The international MR Imaging in MS collaboration has characterized the different MRI appearances of TDLs into four types: ring-enhancing, infiltrative, megacystic and Baló-like subtypes. See figures 10.6(a)–(d).

TDLs can present as single or multiple lesions and might appear simultaneously at onset or sequentially. Most patients follow the typical course of MS, even though a small group develops relapsing TDL. MRI findings that support TDL include open-ring contrast enhancing, minimum to moderate edema and mass effect for size, a rim of T2 hypointensity, peripheral hypointensity on ADC maps at the lesion edge, and venular enhancement [25].

There is usually a paucity of perilesional edema, and lower cerebral blood volume in at perfusion imaging. Also, tumefactive demyelinating lesions are inflammatory processes and for this reason they contain a higher quantity of water than many tumors, which translates into lower attenuation in computed tomography (CT) and higher signal intensity on T2-W images. Lesions do not always produce a proportional mass effect—'nontumefactive' TDL—thus, the term tumefactive can be a misnomer.

The changes in DW imaging evolve rapidly, in the range of a few days, which is in contrast to the more stable findings in patients with tumors or abscesses. Additionally, gliomas or brain metastases have no ADC restriction and abscesses usually display central rather than peripheral restriction.

Magnetic resonance spectroscopy (MRS) is a promising technique for the detection of lesions. Increased glutamate–glutamine peaks on MRS with short echo times seems to be in favor of the diagnosis of TDLs, and are not typically seen with aggressive neoplastic brain lesions. An increased ratio of CHO (choline) to NAA on MRS with short or intermediate echo time is usually observed in TDLs. MR spectroscopy might show elevated choline or lactate peaks with very high inflammatory activity, but this is a nonspecific sign and can also be seen in tumors.

CT-PET seems to be a useful tool in helping to differentiate between TDLs and neoplasms, as neoplasms have greater metabolic activity than TDLs. However, some inflammatory diseases, such as neurosarcoidosis, might also be hypermetabolic on CT-PET and can in this way mimic TDL. A combination of MR spectroscopy and CT-PET might prove to be useful in the future and ongoing studies are producing promising results [26].

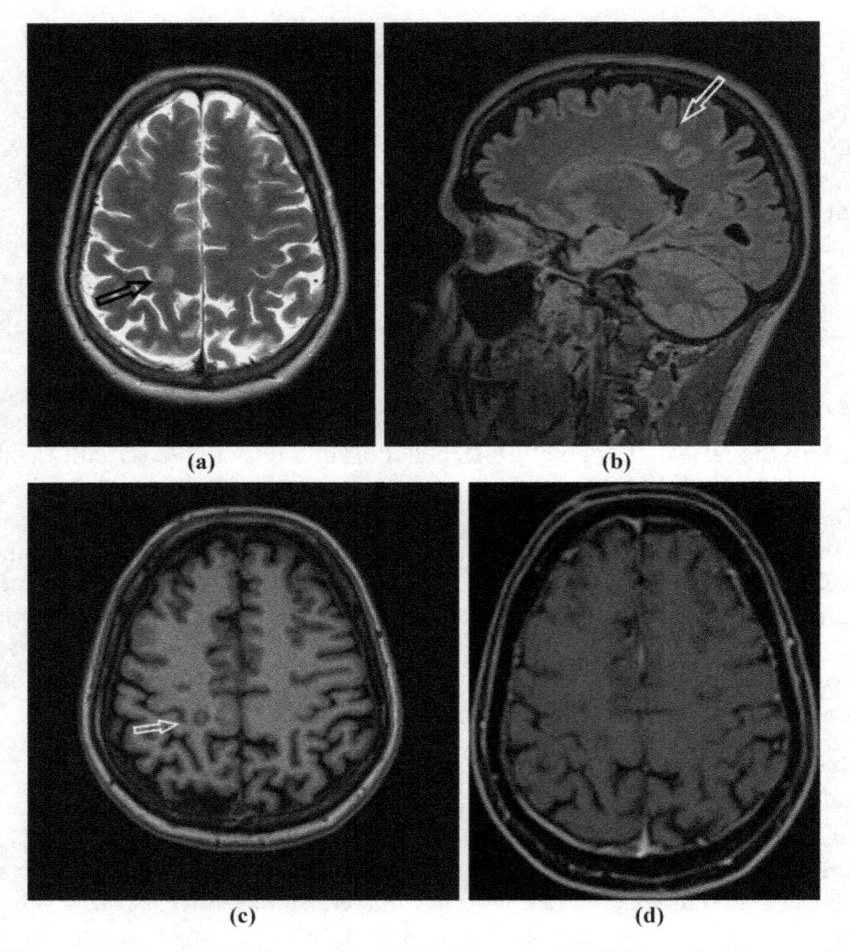

Figure 10.6. A pseudotumor in a 39-year-old woman with suspected MS (the patient was revealed to be affected by Vogt Koyanagi Harada syndrome). Axial T2 (a) and sagittal FLAIR (b) images show a focal solitary lesion, 1 cm in diameter, located in the white matter of the right centrum semiovale. (c) An axial T1 image shows the faint hypointensity of the lesion. (d) Axial T1 after gadolinium contrast administration: the lesion does not show any enhancement.

Follow-up MR studies, particularly after immunosuppressive treatment, frequently demonstrates a reduction in the size and number of lesions [27].

References

[1] Van der Knaap M S *et al* 1992 ^{1}H and ^{31}P MRS of the brain in degenerative cerebral disorders *Ann. Neurol.* **31** 202–11

[2] Polman C H *et al* 2011 Diagnostic criteria for multiple sclerosis: 2010 revisions to the McDonald criteria *Ann. Neurol.* **69** 292–302

[3] Montalban X *et al* 2010 MRI criteria for MS in patients with clinically isolated syndromes *Neurology* **74** 427–34

[4] Filippi M and Rocca M A 2011 MR imaging of multiple sclerosis *Radiology* **259** 659–81

[5] Reimer P *et al* 2010 *Multiple Sclerosis in Clinical MR Imaging* 3rd edn (Berlin: Springer)
[6] Dawson K T 1916 The histology of multiple sclerosis *Trans. R. Soc. Edinb.* **50** 517–740
[7] Filippi M and Rocca M A 2007 Conventional MRI in multiple sclerosis *J. Neuroimaging* **17** 3S–9S
[8] Geurts J J *et al* 2005 Intracortical lesions in multiple sclerosis: improved detection with 3D double inversion-recovery MR imaging *Radiology* **236** 254–60
[9] Nelson F *et al* 2007 Improved identification of intracortical lesions in multiple sclerosis with phase-sensitive inversion recovery in combination with fast double inversion recovery MR imaging *AJNR Am. J. Neuroradiol.* **28** 1645–9
[10] Nelson F *et al* 2008 3D MPRAGE improves classification of cortical lesions in multiple sclerosis *Mult. Scler.* **14** 1214–9
[11] Chen J J *et al* 2016 MRI differential diagnosis of suspected multiple sclerosis *Clin. Radiol.* **71** 815–27
[12] Stankiewicz J *et al* 2007 Iron in chronic brain disorders: imaging and neurotherapeutic implications *Neurotherapeutics* **4** 371–86
[13] Haacke E M *et al* 2010 Iron stores and cerebral veins in MS studied by susceptibility weighted imaging *Int. Angiol.* **29** 149–57
[14] Yousem D M and Grossman R I 2010 *Neuroradiology: The Requisites* 3rd edn (Philadelphia, PA: Mosby)
[15] Hardy T A *et al* 2016 Atypical inflammatory demyelinating syndromes of the CNS *Lancet Neurol.* **15** 967–81
[16] Yonezu T *et al* 2014 'Bright spotty lesions' on spinal magnetic resonance imaging differentiate neuromyelitis optica from multiple sclerosis *Mult. Scler.* **20** 331–7
[17] Kister I *et al* 2013 Ultrahigh-field MR (7 T) imaging of brain lesions in neuromyelitis optica *Mult. Scler. Int.* **2013** 398259
[18] Popescu B F and Lucchinetti C F 2012 Pathology of demyelinating diseases *Annu. Rev. Pathol.* **7** 185–217
[19] Tenembaum S *et al* 2002 Acute disseminated encephalomyelitis: a long-term follow-up study of 84 pediatric patients *Neurology* **59** 1224–31
[20] Stadelmann C *et al* 2005 Tissue preconditioning may explain concentric lesions in Baló type of multiple sclerosis *Brain* **128** 979–87
[21] Hardy T A *et al* 2016 Exploring the overlap between multiple sclerosis, tumefactive demyelination and Baló's concentric sclerosis *Mult. Scler.* **22** 986–92
[22] Berger J *et al* 2013 PML diagnostic criteria *Neurology* **80** 1430–8
[23] Cosottini M *et al* 2008 Diffusion-weighted imaging in patients with progressive multifocal leukoencephalopathy *Eur. Radiol.* **18** 1024e30
[24] Siri A *et al* 2015 Isolated tumefactive demyelinating lesions: diagnosis and long-term evolution of 16 patients in a multicentric study *J. Neurol.* **262** 1637–45
[25] Lucchinetti C F *et al* 2008 Clinical and radiographic spectrum of pathologically confirmed tumefactive multiple sclerosis *Brain* **131** 1759–75
[26] Takenaka S *et al* 2011 Metabolic assessment of monofocal acute inflammatory demyelination using MR spectroscopy and 11C-methionine-, 11C-choline-, and 18F-fluorodeoxyglucose-PET *Brain Tumor Pathol.* **28** 229–38
[27] Al-Okaili R N, Krejza J, Wang S, Woo J H and Melhem E R 2006 Advanced MR imaging techniques in the diagnosis of intraaxial brain tumors in adults *RadioGraphics* **26** S173–89

CPSIA information can be obtained
at www.ICGtesting.com
Printed in the USA
JSHW021226121119
2406JS00002B/14